WB105 CUS
✓MM

WB
AEB
CUS

Color Atlas of Emergency Department Procedures

Color Atlas of Emergency Department Procedures

Catherine B. Custalow, MD, PhD
Assistant Professor
Department of Emergency Medicine
University of Virginia
Charlottesville, Virginia

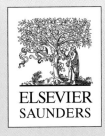

ELSEVIER
SAUNDERS

ELSEVIER
SAUNDERS

The Curtis Center
Independence Square West
Philadelphia, Pa. 19106

COLOR ATLAS OF EMERGENCY DEPARTMENT PROCEDURES   ISBN 0-7216-0447-1
Copyright © 2005, Elsevier Inc.

Notice

Medicine is an ever-changing field. Standard safety precautions must be followed, but as new research and clinical experience broaden our knowledge, changes in treatment and drug therapy may become necessary or appropriate. Readers are advised to check the most current product information provided by the manufacturer of each drug to be administered to verify the recommended dose, the method and duration of administration, and contraindications. It is the responsibility of the treating physician, relying on experience and knowledge of the patient, to determine dosages and the best treatment for each individual patient. Neither the Publisher nor the editor assumes any liability for any injury and/or damage to persons or property arising from this publication.

The Publisher

Library of Congress Cataloging-in-Publication Data

Custalow, Catherine B.
    Color atlas of emergency department procedures / Catherine B. Custalow.—1st ed.
       p. ; cm.
    ISBN 0-7216-0447-1
    1. Emergency medicine—Handbooks, manuals, etc.   2. Emergency medicine—Atlases.
    3. Medical protocols—Handbooks, manuals, etc.   4. Medical protocols—Atlases.   I. Title.
    [DNLM: 1. Emergency Treatment—methods—Atlases.   2. Emergencies—Atlases. WB 17
    C987c 2005]
    RC86.8.C878 2005
    616.02′5—dc22
                                                                 2004046678

Acquisitions Editor: *Todd Hummel*
Developmental Editor: *Carla Holloway*
Project Manager: *Joan Nikelsky*
Book Designer: *Steven Stave*

Printed in China.

Last digit is the print number: 9 8 7 6 5 4 3 2 1

Dedication

To my son Nicholas, and to the memory of my daughter Lauren, both of whom have taught me that the most important things in life are not found in a book.

Foreword

Emergency medicine is all about excellence, but its domain is the entire span of patient care. To that challenge, add the need to act quickly and decisively. Indeed, the measure of time that the emergency physician has to prepare correlates inversely with the desperateness of the situation. As for procedures, Murphy's law still prevails. The rarity of performing a technical task is in lockstep with the criticality of the procedure. Although the emergency physician is summoned the least often to undertake a cricothyroidotomy or thoracotomy, it is always under the most grave circumstances. Finally, the amount of time that passes between performances of such tasks can be substantial. To hone and then maintain procedural skills at the ready is daunting for the most veteran clinician.

The free-throw theory from the sport of basketball offers a simple adage for life. The more you practice, the better you become. But therein lies a vexing dilemma. When it comes to procedures in emergency medicine, the chance to rehearse in a hands-on, real-life fashion can be rare indeed. There is increasing reluctance to seek opportunity on the newly dead. Animal models, postmortem specimens, and bioelectronic equipment are contrivances of the live human condition and of limited availability to most.

Fortunately, the *Color Atlas of Emergency Department Procedures* offers the next best alternative to the actual undertaking of a technique. To begin, each procedure is presented in an identical and logical format. The standard template provides quick-hitting lists of clinical indications, often-overlooked contraindications, potential complications in the aftermath, and an uncluttered set of equipment. The technical stages are laid out in stepwise fashion, with each component accompanied by a relevant color drawing paired with a photograph of the identical anatomy. These features lend themselves to the relaxed study at home or the rapid refresher in the department.

The artwork and photography have been overseen by an experienced anatomist-clinician and, as such, are elegant yet mindful of simplicity and common-sense. The *Atlas* is the quintessential integration of the art and science of medicine and reflects a true labor of love by its author.

The clinician and academician would be well served to read this atlas again and again. It instills a proper approach to the procedure, familiarity in its execution, and confidence in its performance. Why again and again? Because, you never know when next the need will arise.

John A. Marx, M.D.

Preface

Certain emergency department procedures are so rarely performed in clinical practice that physicians may be called upon to complete a life-saving task that they have only read about. I performed my first cricothyroidotomy on a human patient in a rural emergency department the day following my graduation from residency. Following this challenging experience, I realized how indebted I was to my teachers for preparing me for that moment. I also began to appreciate the fact that we can never underestimate the importance of a multifaceted approach to procedural education, including textbooks, atlases, lectures, videotapes, and alternative procedural models to prepare for the uncommon emergencies in clinical practice.

The *Color Atlas of Emergency Department Procedures* represents a novel approach to procedural education. An identical template is used for each chapter. Each procedure is introduced with a brief description and bulleted review of indications, contraindications, complications, and essential equipment. The procedure is presented as a series of ordered steps using a layered approach. Subsequent steps are peeled away, and in this manner the reader progresses logically through the chapter.

Anatomy is an essential foundation for understanding procedures. After many years of teaching anatomy and emergency department procedures, I have been impressed with the importance of having a three-dimensional perspective and a comprehension of the adjacent anatomy so that a procedure can be performed both quickly and competently. In this book, the same perspective and magnification are maintained throughout each step of a procedure so that the reader can remain oriented all along the way.

Each procedural step is illustrated in two ways. First, a color drawing illuminates relevant anatomical structures and their relationship to each new step. Second, a medical photograph provides a realistic clinical view of the step.

The illustrations for this work are intended to provide enough detail so that the reader will understand the relevant anatomy and its relationship to the procedural steps. The celebrated medical illustrator Frank Netter has said: "It is important to achieve a happy medium between complexity and simplification. If the pictures are too complex, they may be difficult and confusing to read; if oversimplified, they may not be adequately definitive or may even be misleading. I have therefore striven for a middle course of realism without the clutter of confusing minutiae" (Netter FM: *Atlas of Human Anatomy*. Hong Kong, CIBA-GEIGY, 1989). This was my intent in this atlas as well.

The written text accompanying each step is purposefully concise to allow the illustrations and photographs to guide the procedural steps. Before actually undertaking any procedure, it is important to have a comprehensive understanding of the details, and I encourage the reader to review each procedure in a more comprehensive text such as Roberts and Hedges' *Clinical Procedures in Emergency Medicine* (4th ed., Philadelphia, WB Saunders, 2004).

This atlas provides a practical reference for many common procedures in the emergency department. It should be a valuable asset to physicians who are learning the rarely performed procedures illustrated herein so that they may rehearse them many times over in their minds. Then, when the occasion demands, the physician will be able to approach the procedure with confidence, assembling the necessary equipment and performing the procedure quickly and competently.

Catherine B. Custalow, MD, PhD

Acknowledgments

Thanks to Anne Olson, senior medical illustrator, and Beth Borchelt, senior medical photographer, from Carolinas Medical Center, who have been with this project from the beginning. Not only have they helped to shape its outcome in so many ways, but they have also made it a joyful effort of the heart.

Thanks also to Nick Lang and Lydia Kibiuk for medical illustrations and to Mike Stevenson and Kevin Custalow for medical photography.

I appreciate Jeff Kline, MD, Katherine Haltiwanger, MD, and Allan Wolfson, MD, for their assistance with content and text review and for their new ideas and constant feedback over the years.

Special thanks to the models who posed for this book, including Jonathan Linko, Katherine Haltiwanger, Mark Heatley, and Nellie Crowder.

Thanks to Todd Hummel, of Elsevier, for his wellspring of patience, grace, and optimism.

And finally, a heart full of gratitude to a respected colleague and friend for saving my life in Chicago, without whom none of this would have been possible. And my acknowledgments to Calvin and Orlando, wherever they are now, for making me realize that every new day of my life is a gift.

Contents

Arthrocentesis

Description:
Arthrocentesis is a procedure in which a needle is inserted into a joint space to obtain synovial fluid.

Indications:
- To diagnose the cause of a joint effusion
- For pain relief from effusion or hemarthrosis

Contraindications:
- Injection through an area of cellulitis
- Bleeding diathesis

Complications:
- Bleeding
- Infection
- Damage to the articular surface of the joint
- Technical failure such as breakage of the needle

Equipment:
A. 10-cc syringe with 19-gauge needle for entering the joint
B. 3-cc or 5-cc syringe with 27-gauge needle for anesthetizing the skin
C. 1% or 2% lidocaine solution

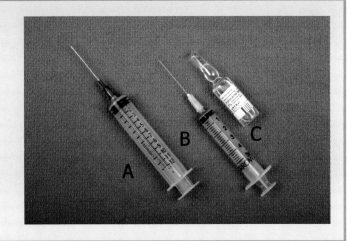

Arthrocentesis of the Knee

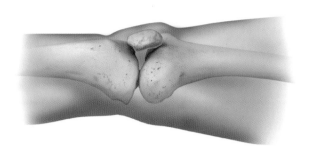
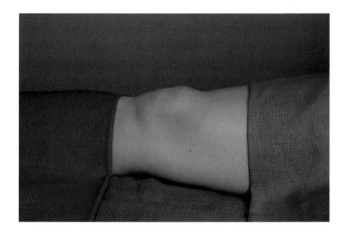

Step 1. Place the patient supine with the knee extended.

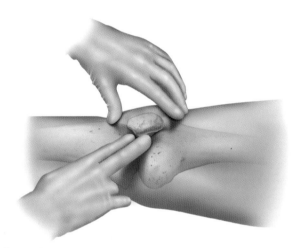
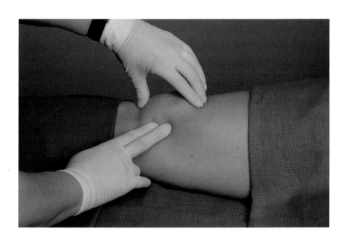

Step 2. Palpate the borders of the patella and select a medial or lateral approach.

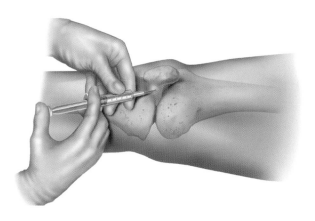

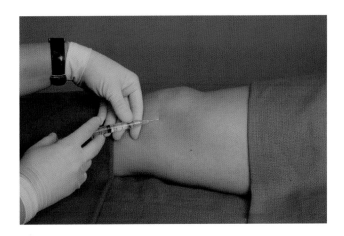

Step 3. Anesthetize the skin.

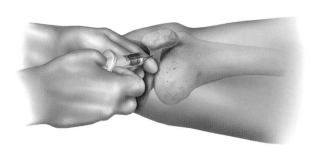

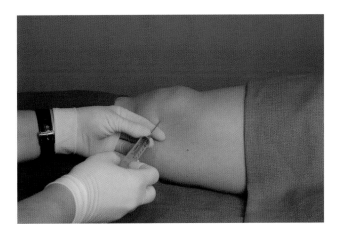

Step 4. Enter the skin between the patella and the joint midway between the superior and inferior poles of the patella.

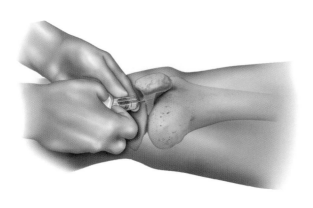

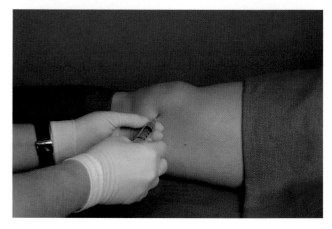

Step 5. Aspirate gently on the syringe while advancing the needle into the joint. Withdraw synovial fluid into the syringe.

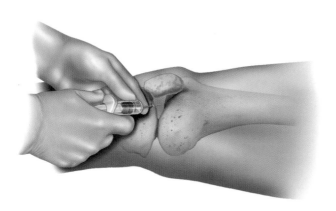

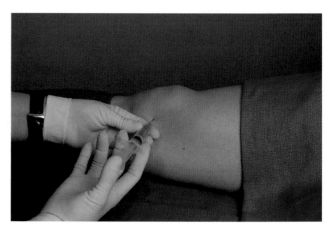

Step 6. If necessary, inject anesthetic solution into the joint for pain relief.

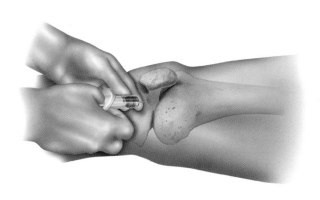
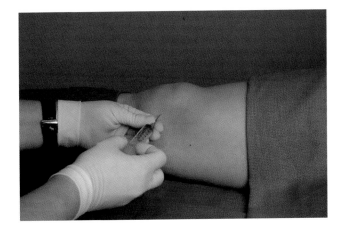

Step 7. Withdraw the needle.

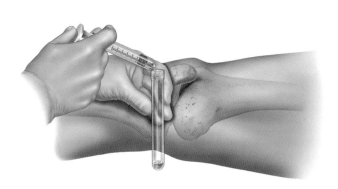
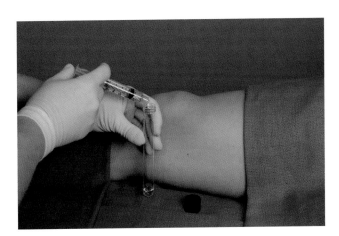

Step 8. Send the synovial fluid to the laboratory for analysis.

Arthrocentesis of the Ankle

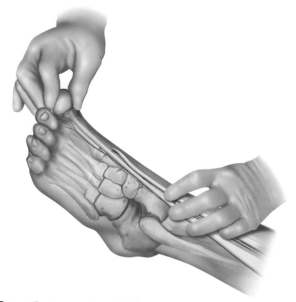 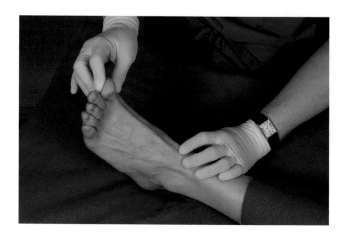

Step 1. Locate the tibialis anterior and extensor hallucis longus tendons by having the patient dorsiflex the foot and raise the toe.

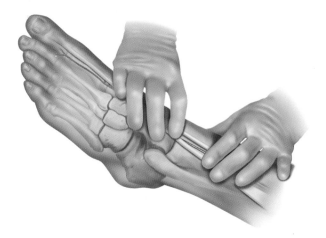 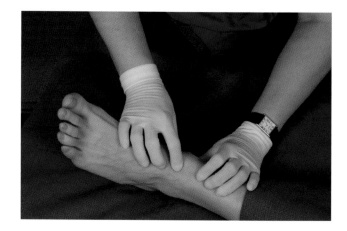

Step 2. Identify the joint line between the tibia and talus.

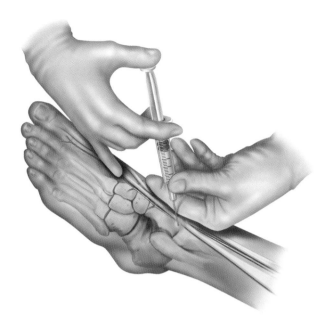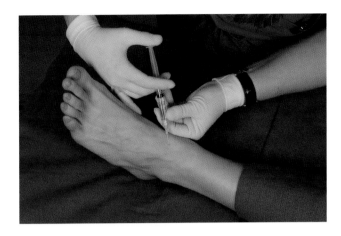

Step 3. Anesthetize the skin overlying the joint.

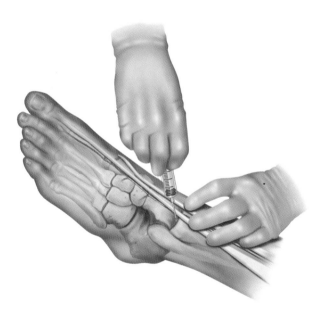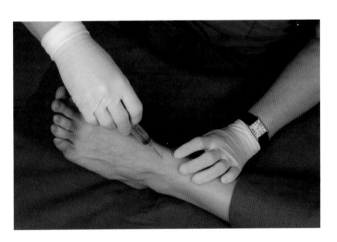

Step 4. Direct the needle perpendicular to the skin between the tibia and talus, lateral to the tendons. Avoid the artery and any visible veins.

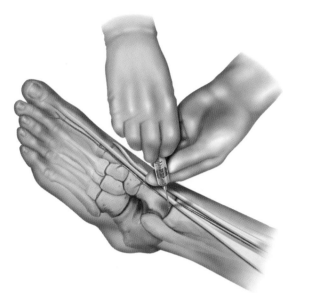

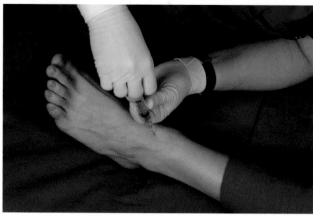

Step 5. Aspirate gently on the syringe while advancing the needle into the joint. Withdraw synovial fluid into the syringe.

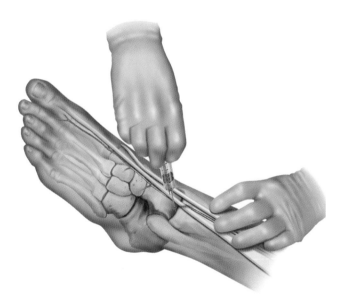

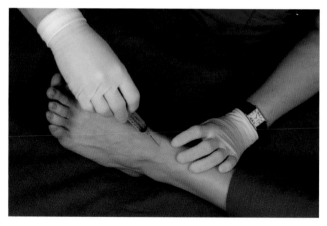

Step 6. Withdraw the needle.

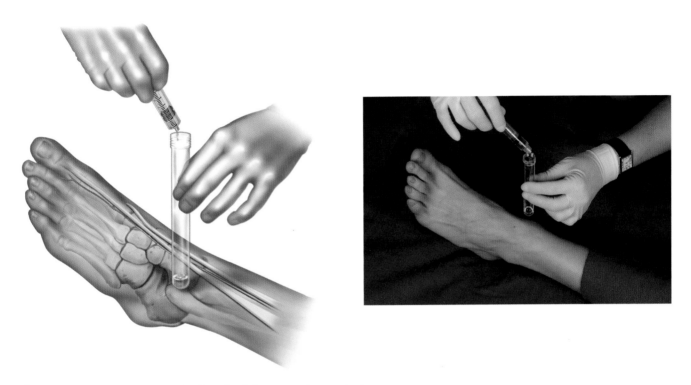

Step 7. Send the synovial fluid to the laboratory for analysis.

Arthrocentesis of the Elbow

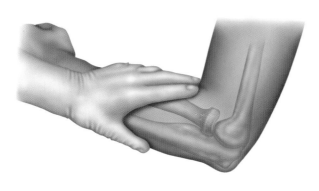

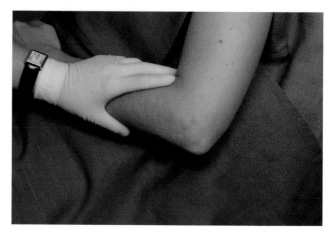

Step 1. Stabilize the elbow joint at a 90-degree angle with the thumb pointing up.

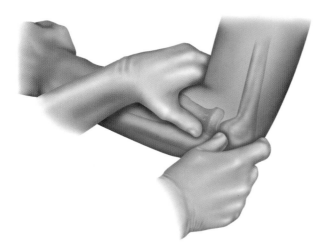

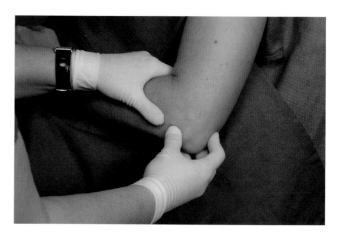

Step 2. Palpate the soft triangle between the radial head, the olecranon, and the lateral epicondyle of the humerus.

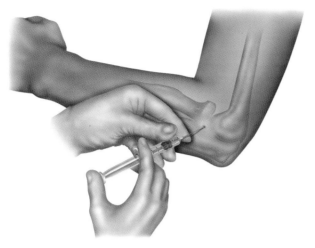
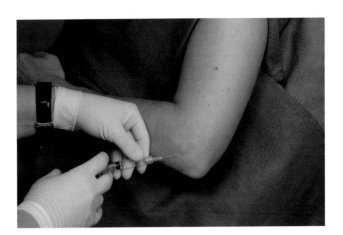

Step 3. Anesthetize the skin overlying the joint.

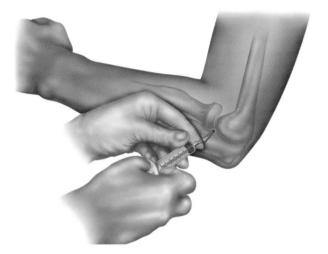
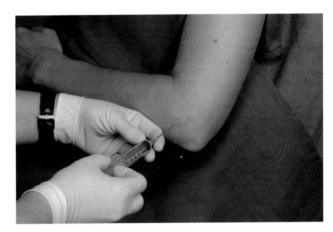

Step 4. Enter the joint from the lateral side.

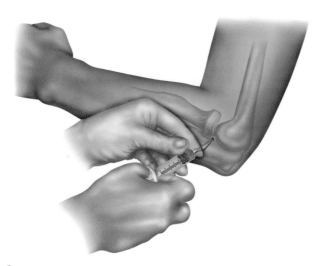
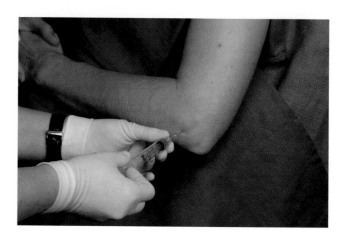

Step 5. Aspirate gently on the syringe while advancing the needle into the joint. Withdraw synovial fluid into the syringe.

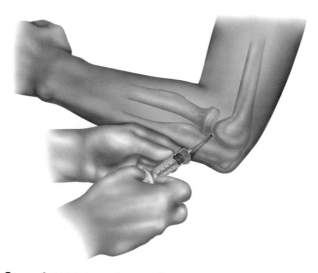
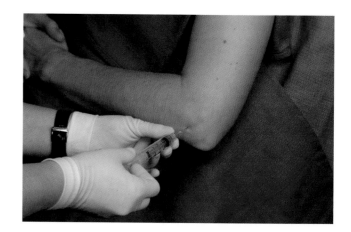

Step 6. Withdraw the needle.

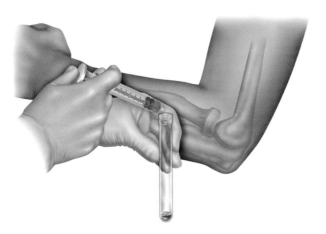 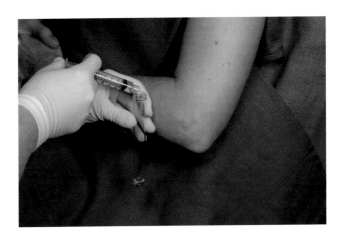

Step 7. Send the synovial fluid to the laboratory for analysis.

Central Vein Catheterization

Description:
Central vein catheterization is a procedure in which a central vein is cannulated percutaneously.

Indications:
- Emergency vascular access
- Inability to obtain peripheral intravenous (IV) access
- Measurement of central venous pressure
- Access for transvenous pacemaker

Contraindications:
- Bleeding diathesis
- Uncooperative patient
- Overlying cellulitis
- Trauma proximate to the area of the cannulation site

Complications:
- Bleeding
- Infection
- Pneumothorax
- Hemothorax
- Pericardial tamponade
- Venous thrombosis
- Lost guidewire
- Catheter embolism
- Injury to nerves

Equipment:
- **A.** 1% lidocaine, syringe, and needle for anesthetizing skin
- **B.** Introducer needle and syringe
- **C.** Guidewire and holder
- **D.** Scalpel—No. 11 blade
- **E.** Tissue dilator
- **F.** Central venous catheter
- **G.** Plastic skin attachments
- **H.** Silk suture
- **I.** IV tubing

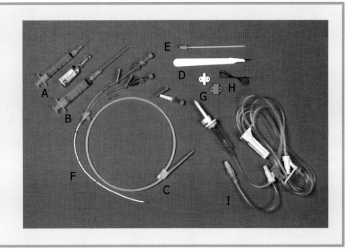

Subclavian Vein Catheterization

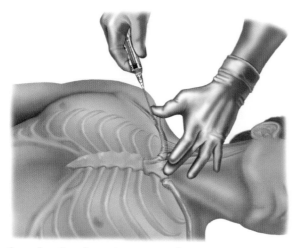

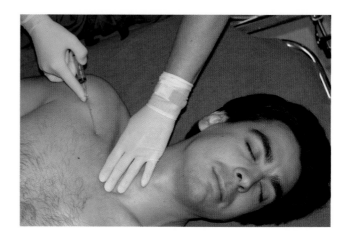

Infraclavicular Approach

Step 1. Insert the needle just inferior to the clavicle between the middle and lateral thirds of the clavicle. Direct the needle medially and slightly cephalad. Aim toward the suprasternal notch.

Steps 2 through 15. Seldinger technique as described later on.

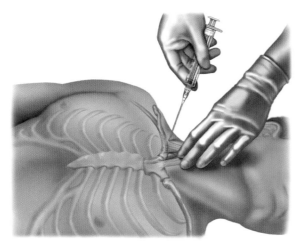

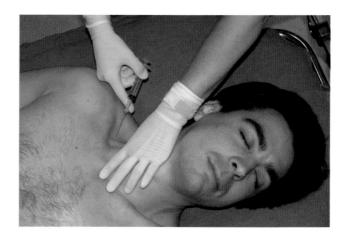

Supraclavicular Approach

Step 1. Insert the needle 1 cm above the clavicle and 1 cm lateral to the clavicular head of the sternocleidomastoid muscle. Aim the needle toward the suprasternal notch or the contralateral nipple.

Steps 2 through 15. Seldinger technique as described later on.

Internal Jugular Vein Catheterization

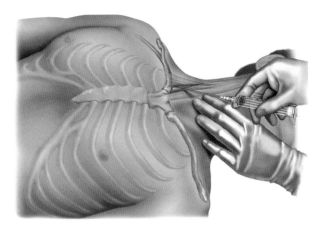

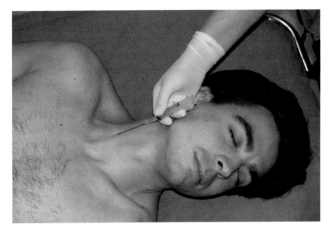

Central Approach

Step 1. Identify a triangle formed by the sternal head of the sternocleidomastoid muscle, the clavicular head of the sternocleidomastoid muscle, and the clavicle. Insert the needle at the apex of the triangle at a 30–45 degree angle to the skin. Aim toward the ipsilateral nipple.

Steps 2 through 15. Seldinger technique as described later on.

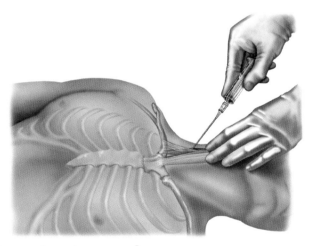

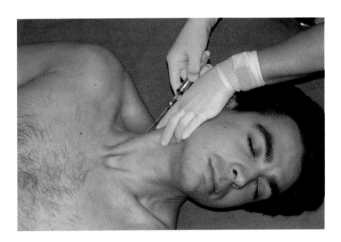

Posterior Approach

Step 1. Identify the posterior border of the sternocleidomastoid muscle. Insert the needle at the posterior edge of the sternocleidomastoid muscle, one third of the distance from the clavicle to the mastoid. Direct the needle under the muscle toward the suprasternal notch.

Steps 2 through 15. Seldinger technique as described later on.

Femoral Vein Catheterization

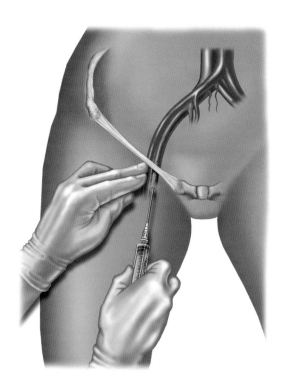

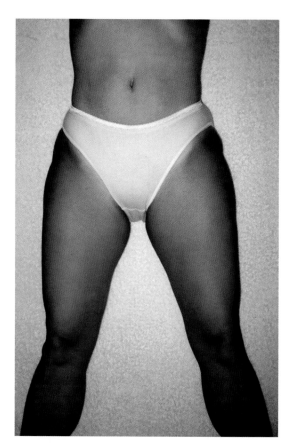

Step 1. Palpate the femoral artery pulse just inferior to the inguinal ligament, midway between the anterior superior iliac spine and the pubic tubercle. Insert the needle into the femoral canal at a 45-degree angle to the skin, just medial to the femoral pulse.

Steps 2 through 15. Seldinger technique as described later on.

Seldinger Technique (Subclavian Infraclavicular Approach)

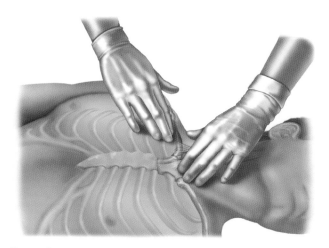

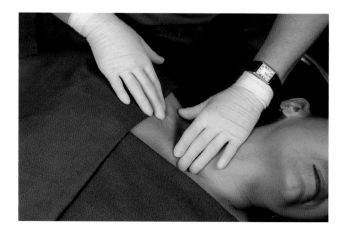

Step 1. Identify the anatomic landmarks.

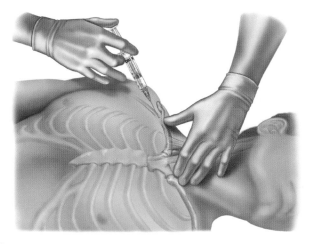 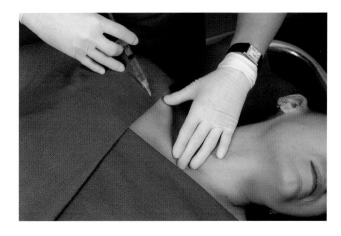

Step 2. Anesthetize the skin and subcutaneous tissues with 1% lidocaine.

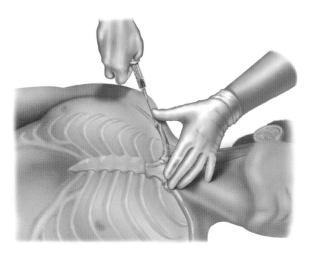 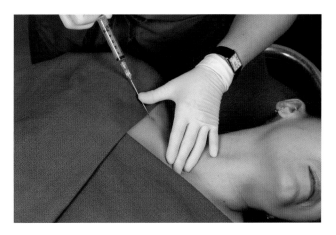

Step 3. Insert the introducer needle while gently aspirating for blood.

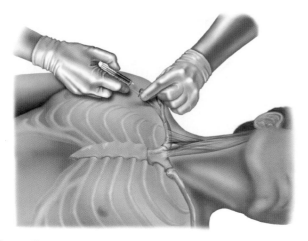 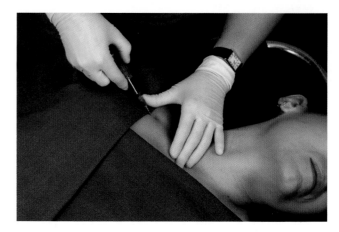

Step 4. Once venous blood is being withdrawn easily, remove the syringe.

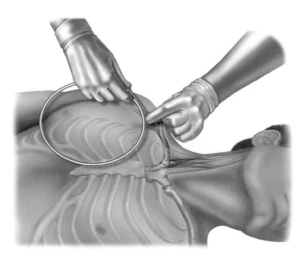 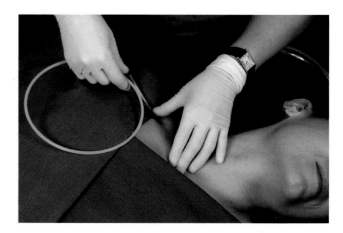

Step 5. Pass the flexible guidewire through the needle into the vessel.

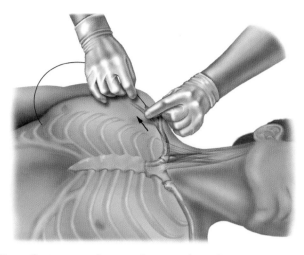

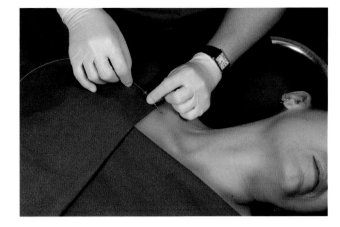

Step 6. Remove the needle over the wire.

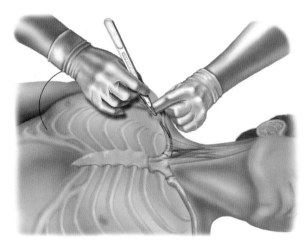

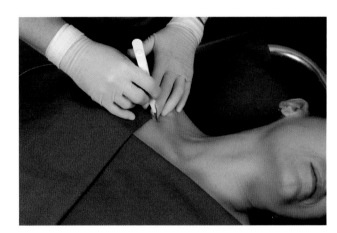

Step 7. Make a small skin incision at the site of the guidewire.

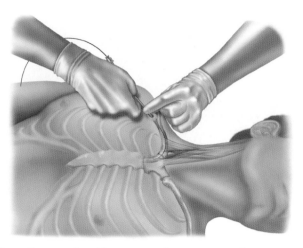 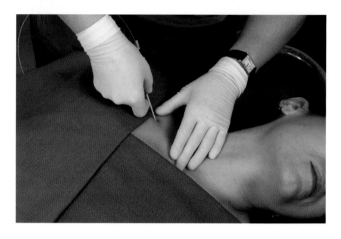

Step 8. Pass the dilator over the wire to make a tunnel through the subcutaneous tissues.

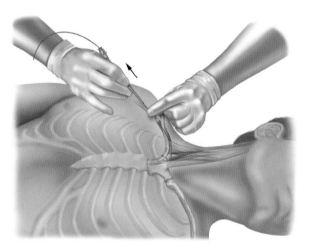 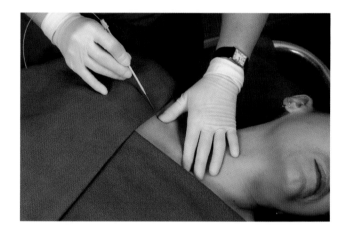

Step 9. Remove the dilator, keeping the guidewire in place.

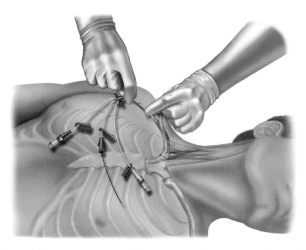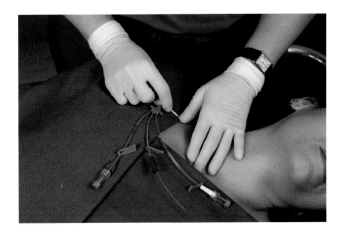

Step 10. Pass the central venous catheter over the guidewire into the vessel.

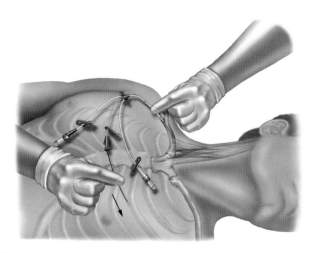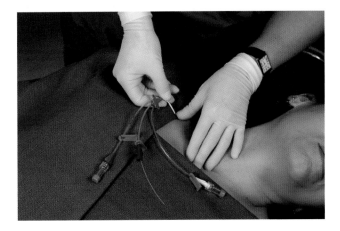

Step 11. Remove the guidewire.

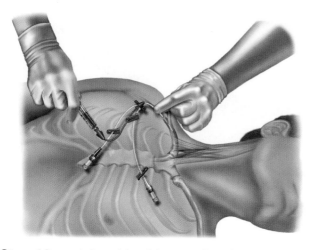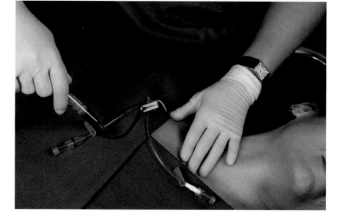

Step 12. Withdraw blood from each catheter port.

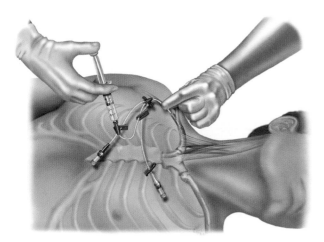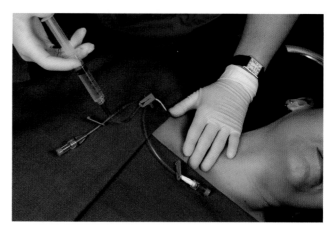

Step 13. Flush each catheter port with sterile saline and cover each port with a Luer-Lok cap.

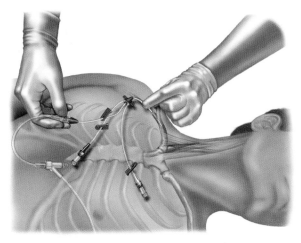
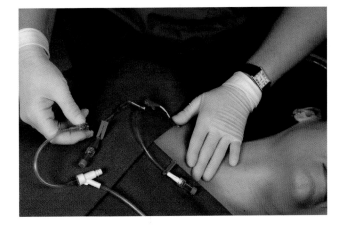

Step 14. Attach the catheter to the IV tubing.

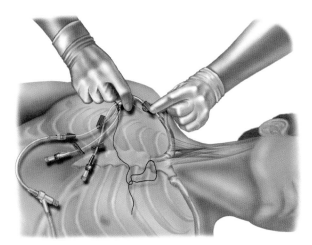
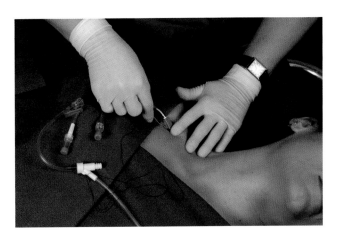

Step 15. Suture the catheter into place, using the blue and white skin attachment collars.

Compartment Pressure Measurement

Description:
Measurement of compartment pressure is a procedure in which the fascial compartment pressure is measured by inserting a needle with an attached manometer into a compartment of the arm or leg.

Indications:
- An extremity injury such as fracture, burn, prolonged compression or crush in which elevated compartment pressure is suspected
- Clinical findings present at varying degrees of severity, including
  - Pain, especially when out of proportion to clinical findings
  - Paresthesia
  - Paresis
  - Pulselessness
  - Palpable tenseness of the compartment
  - Pallor

Contraindications:
- Overlying skin infection
- Bleeding diathesis

Complications:
- Pain
- Bleeding
- Infection
- Damage to neurovascular structures within the compartment

Equipment:

A. Stryker intracompartmental pressure monitor

B. Disposable quick-pressure monitor system assembly, including 3-cc syringe filled with sterile saline and 18-gauge needle

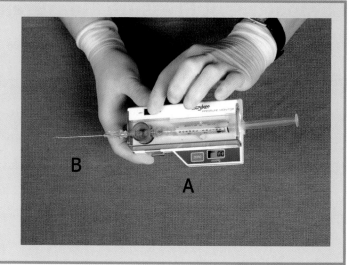

Forearm Compartments

All forearm compartments are entered in the area of the junction of the proximal and middle thirds of the forearm.

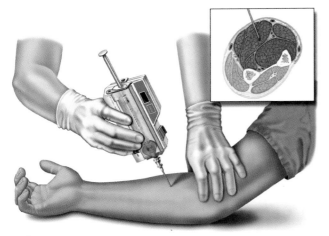

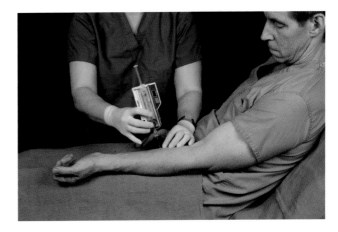

Volar Compartment:

Enter the volar compartment just between the palmaris longus tendon and the radial surface of the ulna. Insert to a depth of 1-2 cm.

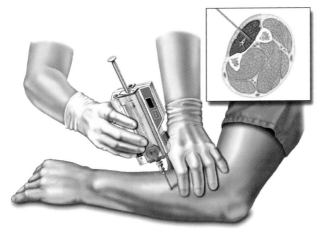

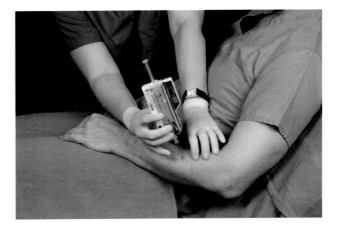

Dorsal Compartment:

Enter the dorsal compartment 1-2 cm lateral to the posterior aspect of the ulna. Insert to a depth of 1-2 cm.

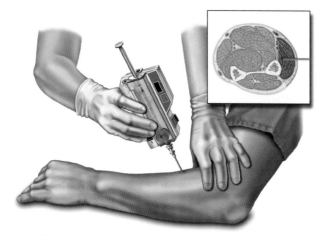 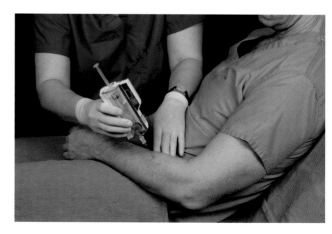

Mobile Wad Compartment:

Enter the mobile wad just lateral to the radius. Insert to a depth of 1-1.5 cm.

Lower Leg Compartments

All lower leg compartments are entered in the area of the junction of the proximal and middle thirds of the lower leg.

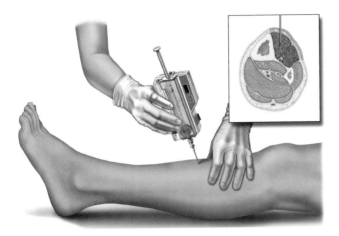 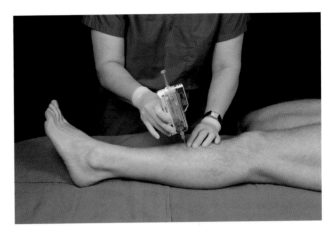

Anterior Compartment:

Enter the anterior compartment 1 cm lateral to the border of the anterior tibia. Insert to a depth of 1-3 cm.

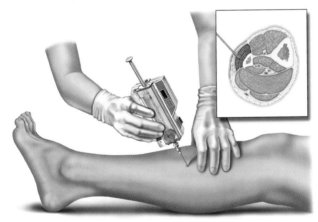 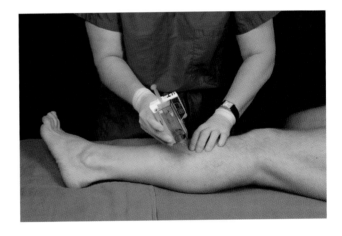

Lateral Compartment:

Enter the lateral compartment at the posterior border of the fibula. Insert to a depth of 1-1.5 cm.

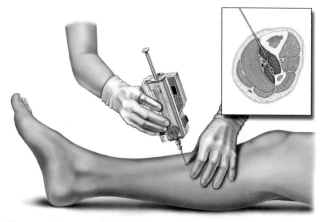
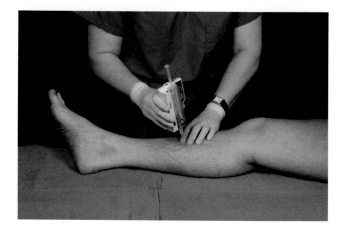

Deep Posterior Compartment:

Enter the deep posterior compartment just posterior to the medial border of the tibia. Insert to a depth of 2-4 cm in the direction of the posterior border of the fibula.

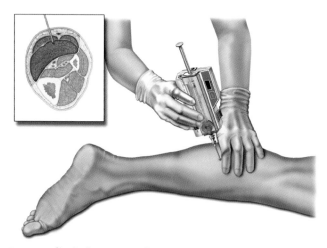
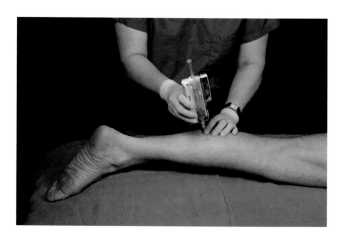

Superficial Posterior Compartment:

Enter the superficial posterior compartment posteriorly directly over the center of the gastrocnemius muscle. Insert to a depth of 1-1.5 cm.

Cricothyroidotomy

Description:
Cricothyroidotomy is a procedure in which a surgical opening is made in the cricothyroid membrane in order to insert an airway.

Indications:
Inability to intubate the patient endotracheally, as in:
- Massive hemorrhage
- Profound emesis
- Laryngospasm
- Airway obstruction due to oropharyngeal edema
- Clenched teeth
- Mass effect from tumor
- Severe facial injuries
- Obstructing foreign body

Contraindications:
Absolute:
- Ability to safely intubate the patient orally or nasally
- Transection of the trachea
- Fracture of the larynx
- Laryngotracheal disruption
Relative:
- Children less than 8 years old
- Bleeding diathesis

Complications:
- Laceration of the cricoid cartilage
- Laceration of the thyroid cartilage
- Laceration of the tracheal rings
- Inadvertent tracheostomy
- False passage into an extratracheal location
- Excessive bleeding
- Cuff leak
- Infection
- Subglottic stenosis

Equipment:

A. Scalpel—No. 11 blade
B. Trousseau dilator
C. Tracheal hook
D. 10-cc syringe
E. Tracheostomy tube (No. 4 or 6 Shiley, cuffed)
F. Obturator
G. Inner cannula
H. Circumferential tie
I. Bag-valve-mask and ventilator tubing

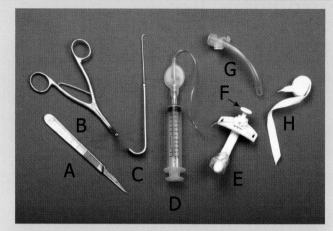

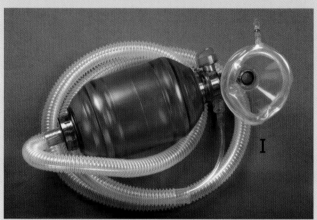

Procedural Steps

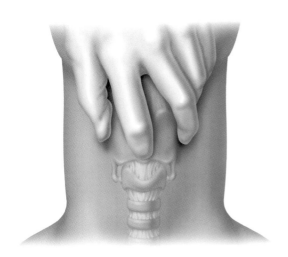

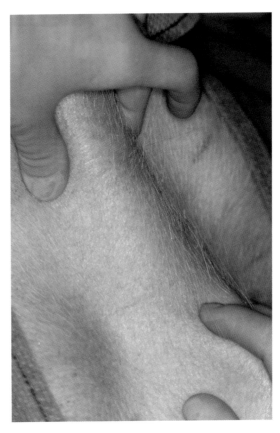

Step 1. Immobilize the larynx and palpate the cricothyroid membrane with the index finger of the non-dominant hand.

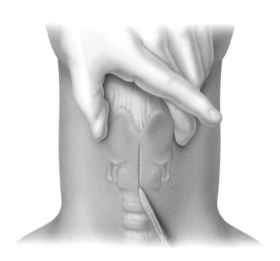

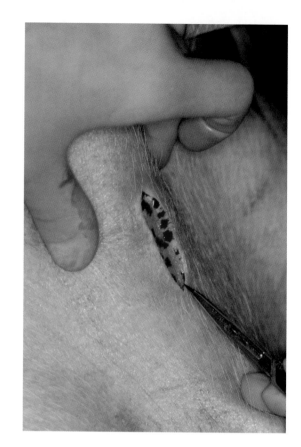

Step 2. Make a midline vertical skin incision, 3-5 cm in length.

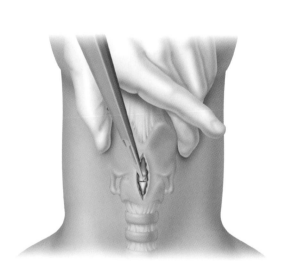

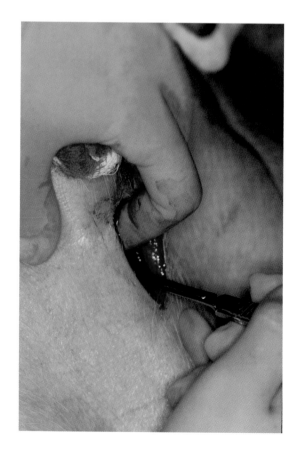

Step 3. Incise the cricothyroid membrane transversely.

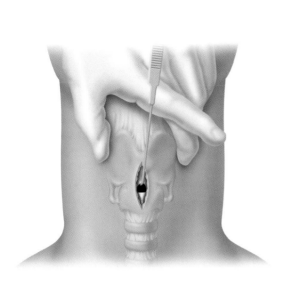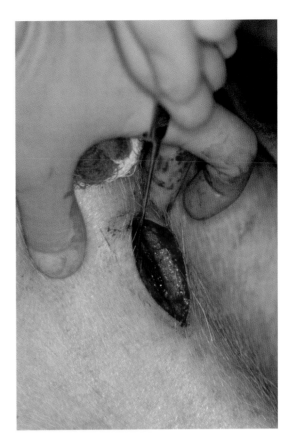

Step 4. Insert the tracheal hook and ask an assistant to provide upward traction.

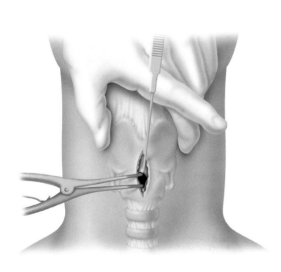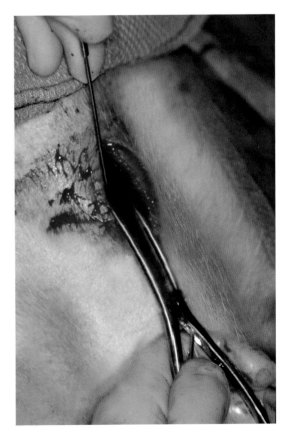

Step 5. Insert the Trousseau dilator and open to expand the incision vertically.

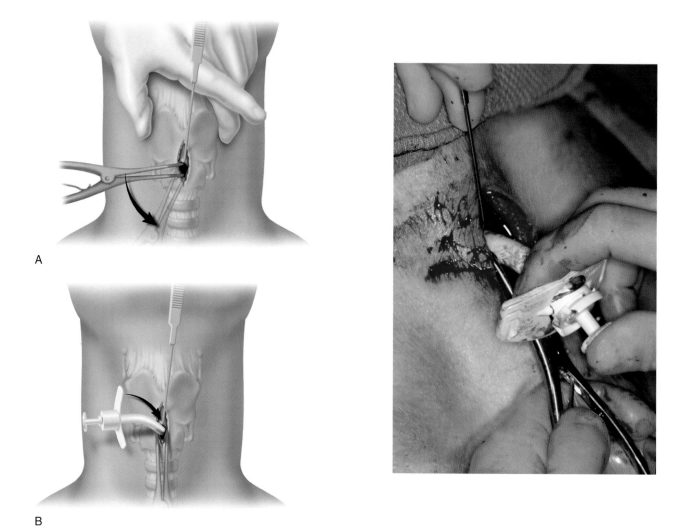

A

B

Step 6. A, Rotate the dilator 90 degrees. **B,** Insert the tracheostomy tube, and advance the tube into the trachea.

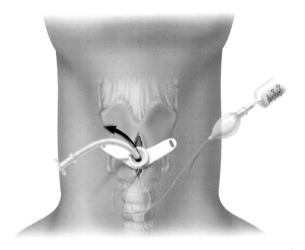

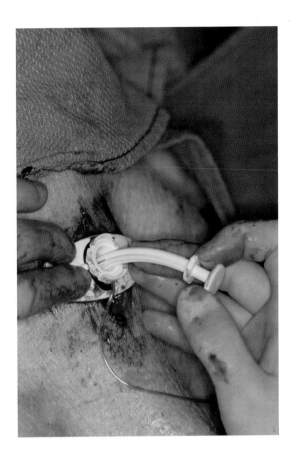

Step 7. Remove the obturator.

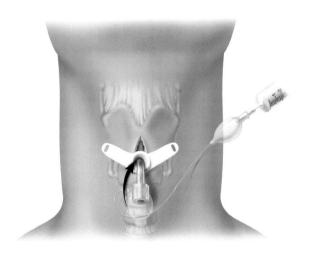

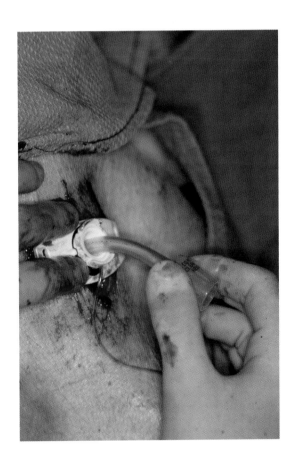

Step 8. Replace the inner cannula and inflate the cuff.

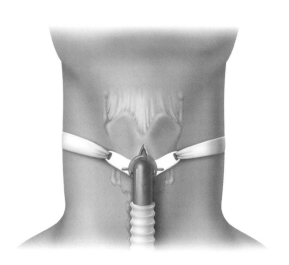

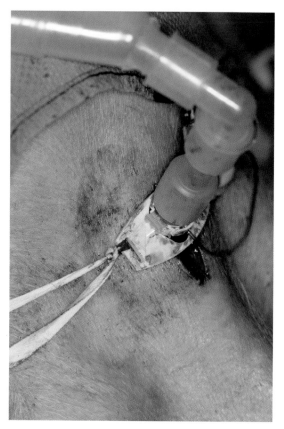

Step 9. Attach ventilator tubing, confirm proper placement, and secure the tube with a circumferential tie around the patient's neck.

Diagnostic Peritoneal Lavage

Description:
Diagnostic peritoneal lavage (DPL) is a procedure in which a catheter is introduced into the peritoneal cavity to evaluate for the presence of blood in the setting of abdominal injury.

Indications:
- Hemodynamic instability in the setting of blunt abdominal trauma
- Suspected blunt abdominal trauma with an unreliable examination
- Stab wound of the abdomen

Contraindications:
Absolute:
- When laparotomy is clinically indicated

Relative:
- Prior abdominal surgery
- Overlying skin infection
- Coagulopathy
- Obesity
- Second or third trimester pregnancy

Complications:
- Bleeding
- Infection
- Rectus sheath hematoma
- Trocar injury to intra-abdominal organs or vessels
- Wound dehiscence
- Incisional hernia

Equipment:

A. Army-Navy retractors
B. Scalpels—No. 11 and 15 blades
C. Curved hemostats
D. Towel clips
E. DPL catheter and trocar
F. IV tubing
G. Right-angle connector
H. 10-cc syringe
I. 1000-mL bag of normal saline or
   lactated Ringer's solution
   (not shown)

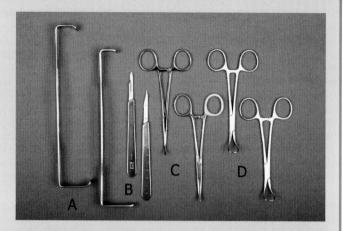

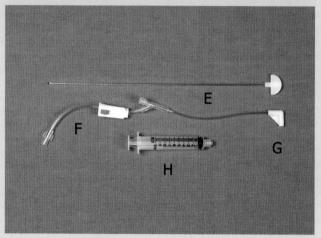

Infraumbilical Approach

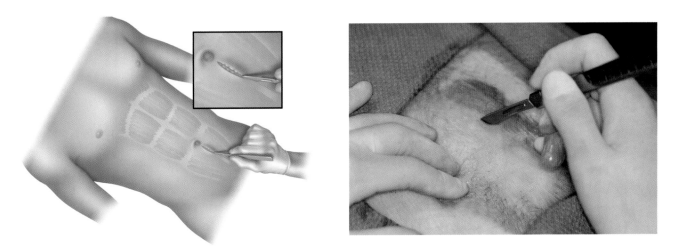

Step 1. Make a 4- to 5-cm vertical skin incision in the midline at the inferior portion of the umbilical ring with a No. 11 scalpel blade.

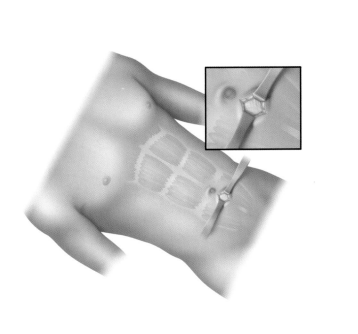

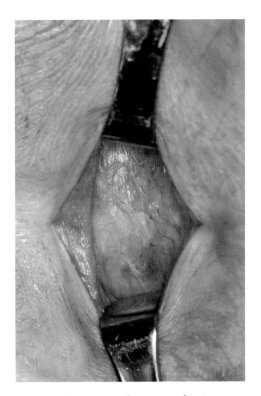

Step 2. Bluntly dissect the subcutaneous tissues with Army-Navy retractors to expose the rectus fascia.

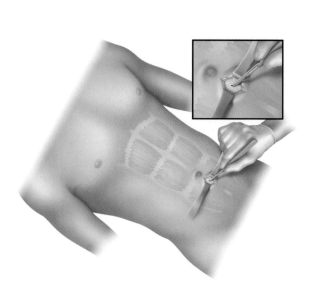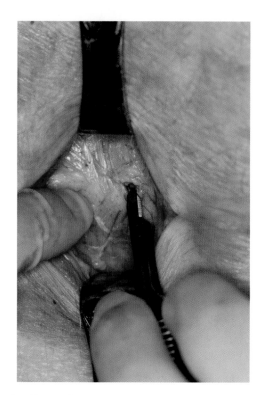

Step 3. Incise the rectus fascia with the No. 15 scalpel blade at the linea alba.

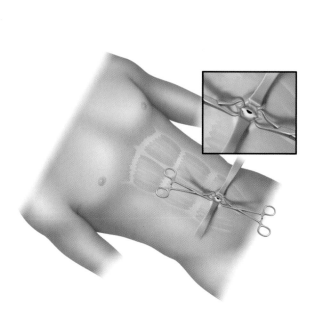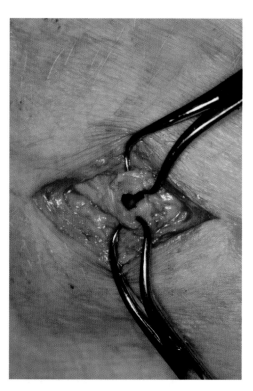

Step 4. Use the towel clips to grasp the rectus fascia and lift it off the peritoneum.

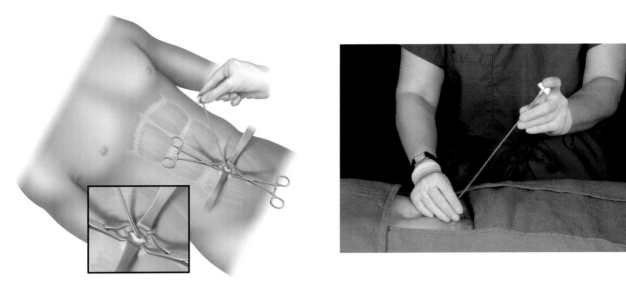

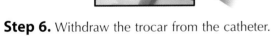

Step 5. Advance the trocar and catheter through the fascial opening into the peritoneum.

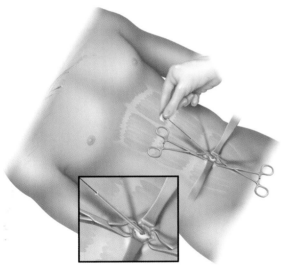

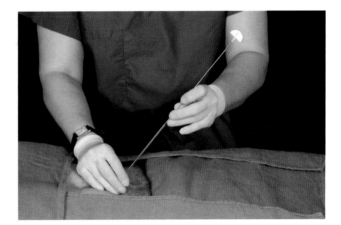

Step 6. Withdraw the trocar from the catheter.

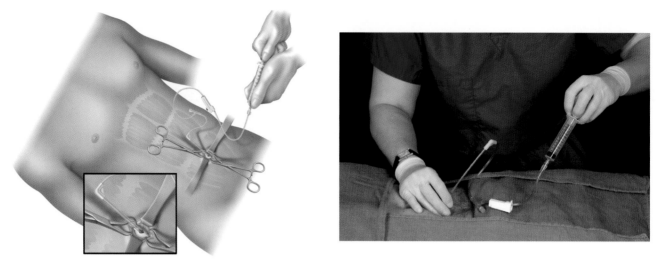

Step 7. Attach the right-angle adapter, extension tubing, and syringe. Attempt aspiration for blood with the syringe.

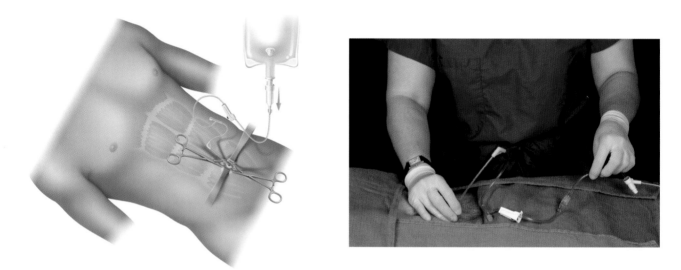

Step 8. If no gross blood is aspirated, instill 1000 mL of normal saline or lactated Ringer's solution into the peritoneal cavity.

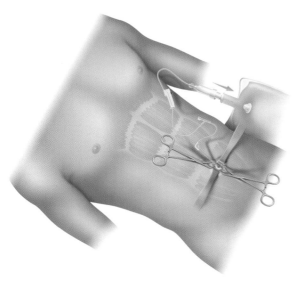
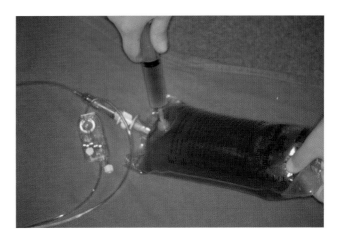

Step 9. Allow the fluid to flow back into the bag by gravity.

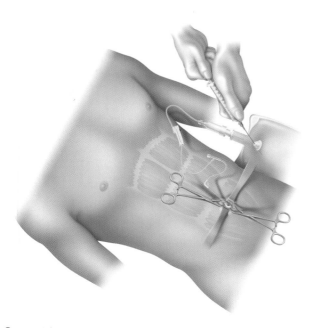
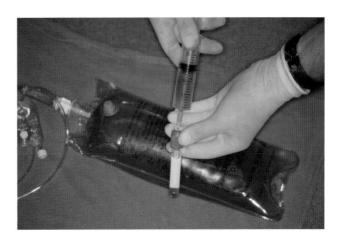

Step 10. Send the effluent to the laboratory for analysis.

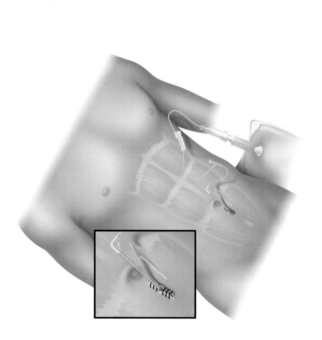

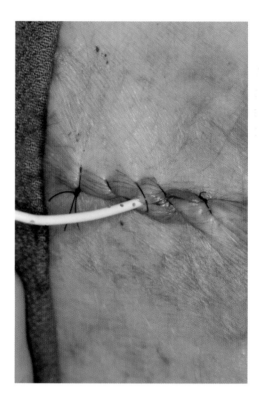

Step 11. Remove the catheter, suture the linea alba, and close the skin primarily. Remove the catheter when the procedure is completed.

Intraosseous Line Placement

Description:
Intraosseous line placement is a procedure in which a specially designed intraosseous needle is placed into the marrow cavity of a long bone for vascular access.

Indication:
For vascular access in children when traditional approaches to intravenous (IV) access are difficult

Contraindications:
Absolute:
- Recent fracture of the bone
- Osteogenesis imperfecta
- Osteoporosis
Relative:
- Overlying skin infection

Complications:
- Cellulitis
- Osteomyelitis
- Extravasation of fluid
- Injury to the growth plate
- Fractures of the bone
- Compartment syndrome
- Fat embolism
- Bacteremia
- Technical problems: breaking the needle or passing through the other side of the bone

Equipment:
A. Intraosseous or bone marrow aspiration needle
B. 10-cc syringe
C. IV tubing

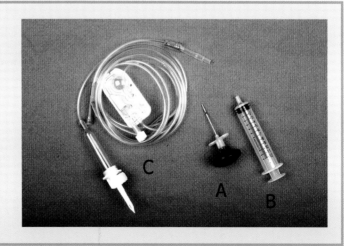

Procedural Steps

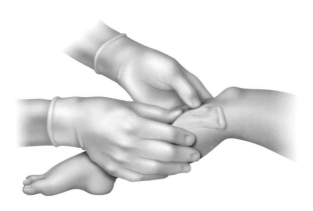 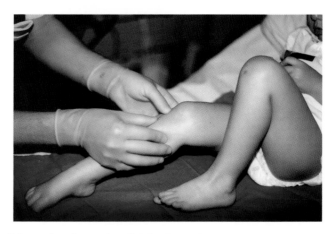

Step 1. Identify the anteromedial surface of the proximal tibia and palpate the tibial tuberosity.

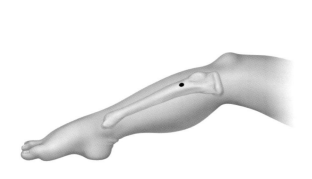 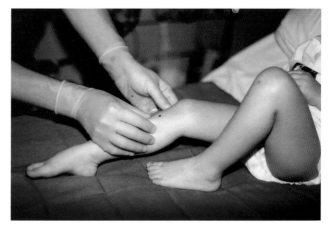

Step 2. The entry site is 1-2 cm distal to the tibial plateau and halfway between the anterior and posterior border of the tibia.

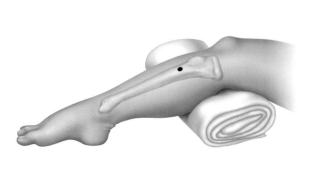
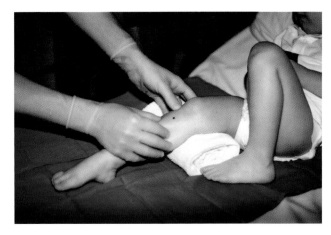

Step 3. Support the patient's leg from underneath with a small towel roll.

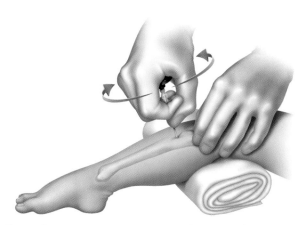
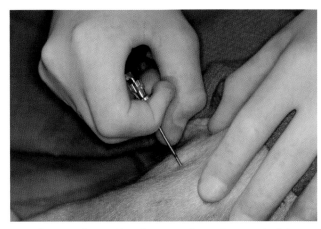

Step 4. Using a twisting rather than a rocking motion, advance the needle until a decrease in resistance is felt.

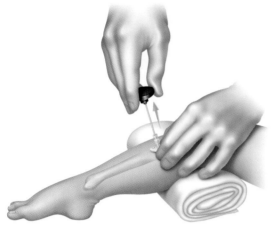

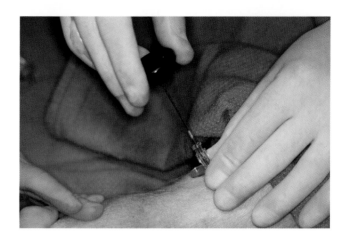

Step 5. Remove the trocar.

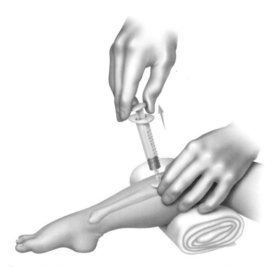

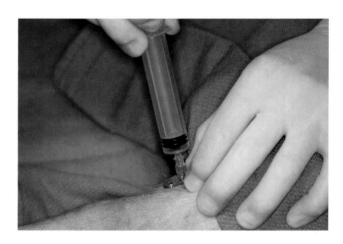

Step 6. Aspirate bone marrow to confirm placement.

Procedural Steps

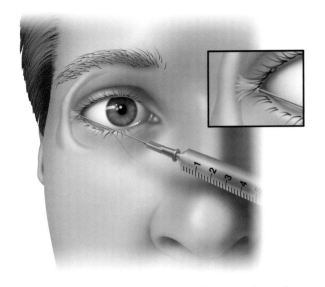

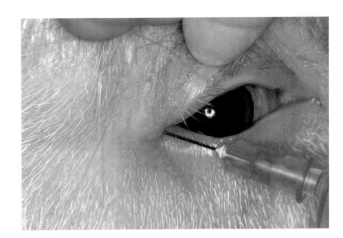

Step 1. Inject 1% lidocaine into the lateral canthus.

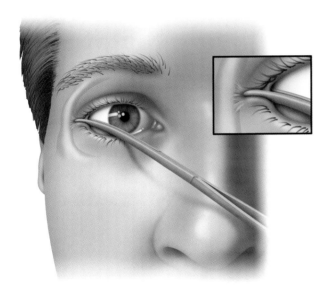

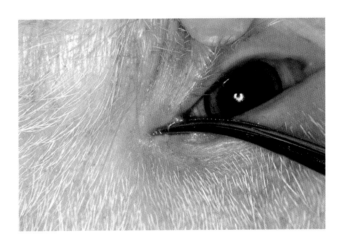

Step 2. Crush the lateral canthus with a small hemostat.

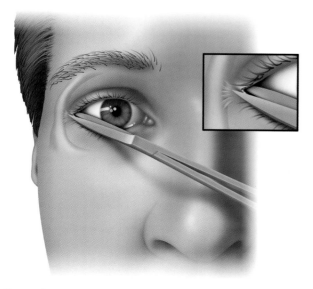 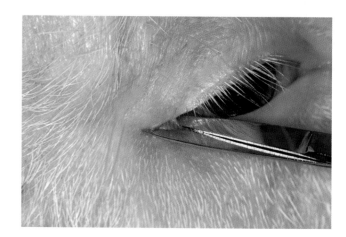

Step 3. Incise the lateral canthus with iris scissors.

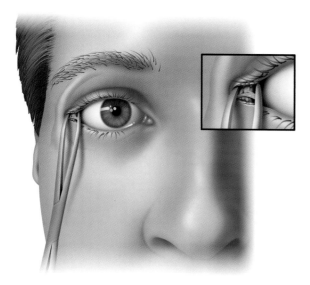 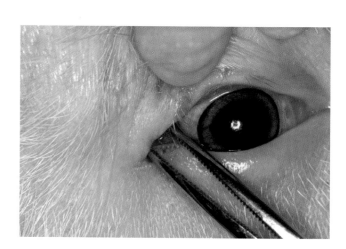

Step 4. Release the canthal ligaments from the orbital rim.

Lumbar Puncture

Description:
Lumbar puncture is a procedure in which a spinal needle is inserted into the lumbar subarachnoid space to obtain cerebrospinal fluid (CSF) for diagnostic or therapeutic purposes.

Indications:
- Suspected central nervous system infection
- Suspected subarachnoid hemorrhage
- Diagnosis and treatment of pseudotumor cerebri

Contraindications:
- Overlying skin or soft-tissue infection
- Significant coagulopathy
- Increased intracranial pressure from mass lesion
- Signs of cerebral herniation
- Spinal cord trauma or compression

Complications:
- Post–lumbar puncture headache
- Infection
- Epidural hematoma
- Backache (local pain)
- Nerve damage
- Epidural abscess
- Diskitis
- Osteomyelitis
- Central nervous system herniation

Equipment:
A. 1% lidocaine solution with needle and syringe
B. Spinal needle with stylet
C. Manometer with three-way stopcock
D. Sterile specimen containers

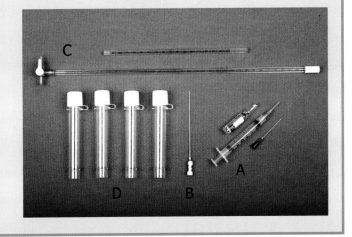

Positioning the Patient

Two positions are commonly used for this procedure—the seated upright position and the lateral decubitus position.

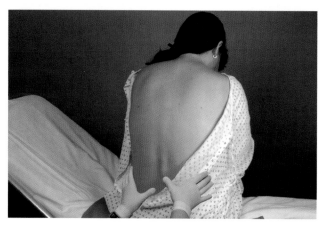

Seated Upright Position

The patient sits on the edge of the bed, bending over a stand or table to open up the intervertebral spaces.

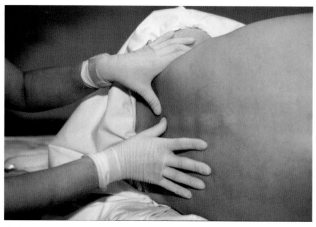

Lateral Decubitus Position

The patient lies on his or her side on a flat bed, flexing the knees and pelvis toward the shoulders to open up the intervertebral spaces. The arms and legs should be held symmetrically. Position the shoulders, pelvis, and back so that they are in a plane perpendicular to the surface of the bed and floor.

Procedural Steps

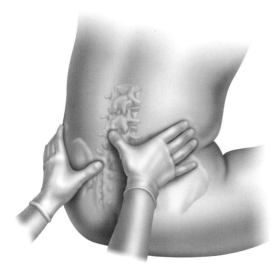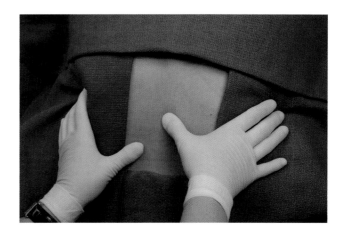

Step 1. Identify the third to fourth lumbar intervertebral space at the top of the iliac crests.

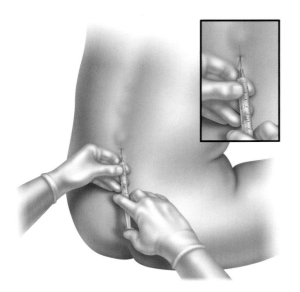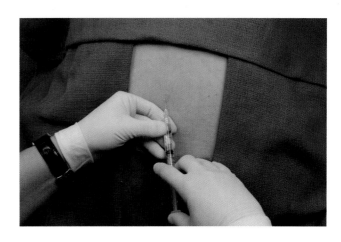

Step 2. Anesthetize the skin and subcutaneous tissues at the injection site.

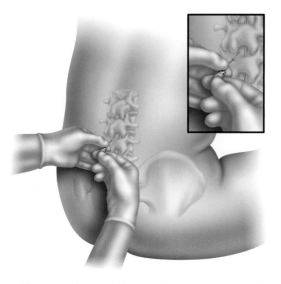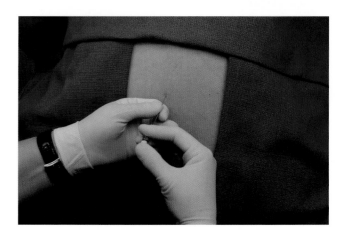

Step 3. Insert the needle into the interspace in the midline and directed slightly cephalad.

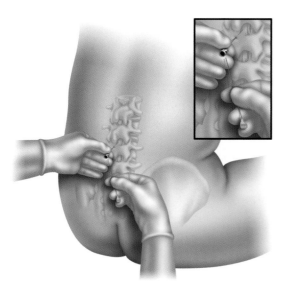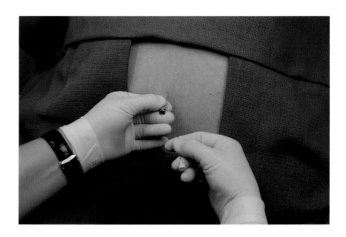

Step 4. Advance the needle slowly, removing the stylet frequently to look for CSF.

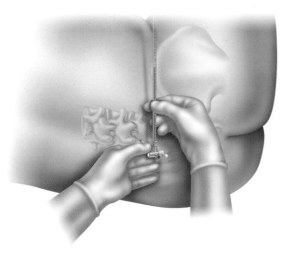 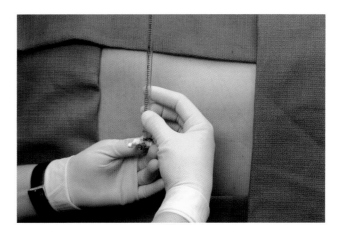

Step 5. Once CSF is seen in the needle, read the opening pressure with the manometer. Place the patient in the lateral decubitus position for this measurement.

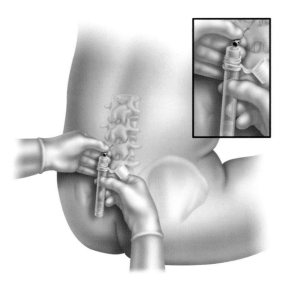 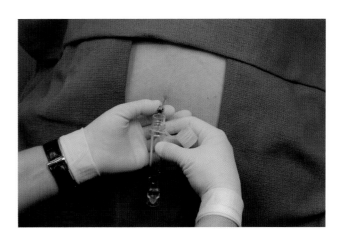

Step 6. Collect CSF for laboratory analysis (approximately 1 cc in each tube).

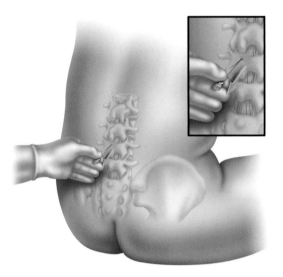 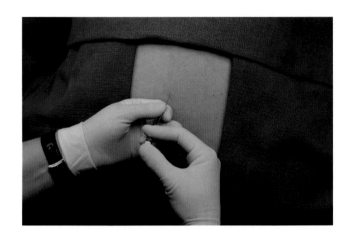

Step 7. Replace the stylet and withdraw both needle and stylet.

Nerve Blocks of the Face, Head, and Oral Cavity

Description:
Nerve blocks of the face, head, and oral cavity are procedures in which anesthetic is injected around a nerve to provide regional anesthesia.

Indications:
- Dental pain
- Dental procedures
- Intraoral procedures
- Repair of facial, ear, or scalp lacerations

Contraindications:
- Injection through an area of infection
- Uncooperative patient
- Bleeding diathesis

Complications:
- Bleeding
- Intravascular injection
- Infection
- Facial nerve injection resulting in temporary paralysis
- Technical failure such as breakage of the needle

Equipment: Dental Syringe

A. Aspirating dental syringe

B. 25- or 27-gauge dental needle

C. Carpule of anesthetic agent—
2% lidocaine with epinephrine
(1:100,000) or
3% mepivacaine or
0.5% bupivacaine

D. Topical anesthetic solution and
cotton-tipped applicator
(not shown)

Equipment: Standard Syringe

E. 3- or 5-cc syringe

F. 25- or 27-gauge standard needle

G. 1% or 2% lidocaine

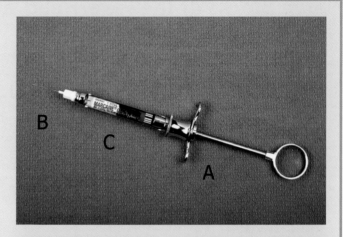

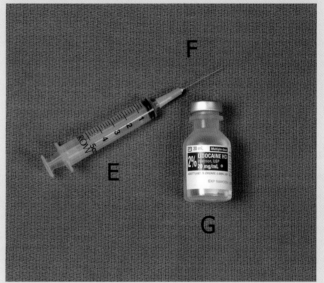

Inferior Alveolar Nerve Block

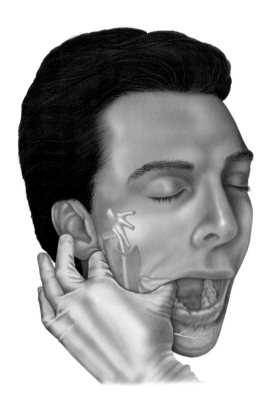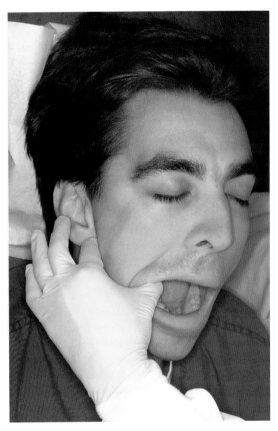

Step 1. Palpate the coronoid process of the mandible with the thumb and forefinger while retracting the cheek laterally.

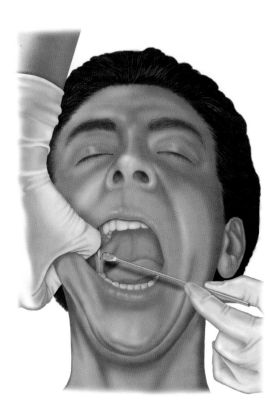
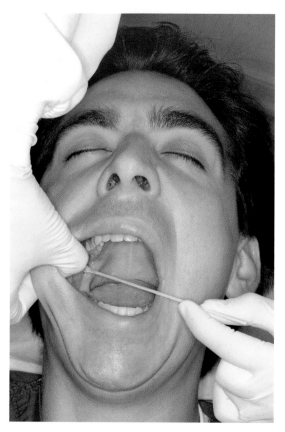

Step 2. Apply topical anesthetic to the mucosa over the intended injection site with a cotton-tipped applicator.

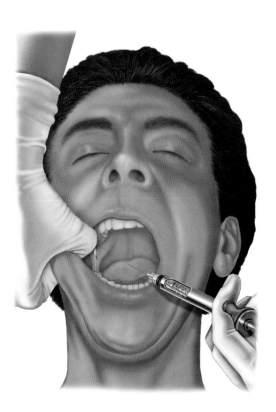
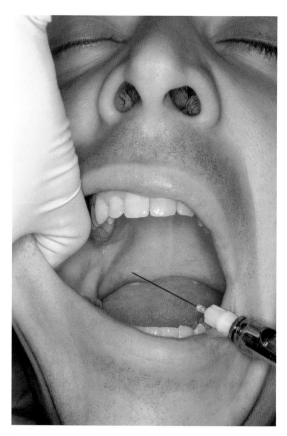

Step 3. Direct the syringe over the first and second premolars of the opposite side and diagonally at the occlusal surfaces of the molars. Identify the site of insertion in the small triangle of tissue posterior to the molars.

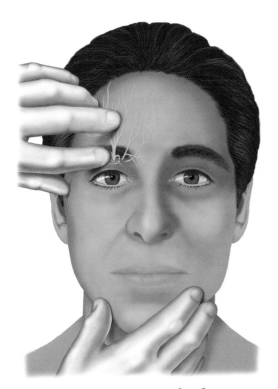
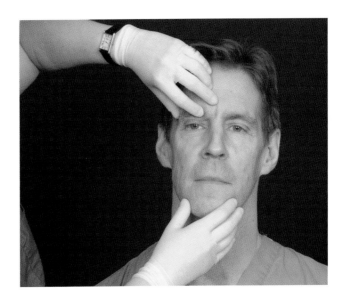

Supraorbital Nerve Block

Step 1. Palpate the supraorbital foramen on the medial aspect of the supraorbital ridge. The foramen will be in a direct line with the pupil when the eye is in the neutral position.

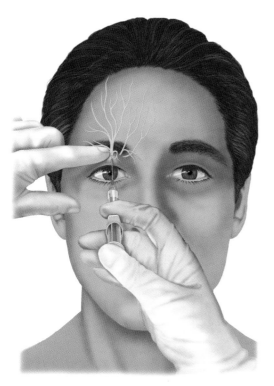
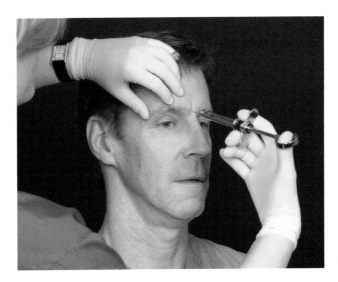

Step 2. Inject 2-3 cc of anesthetic into the area of the supraorbital notch.

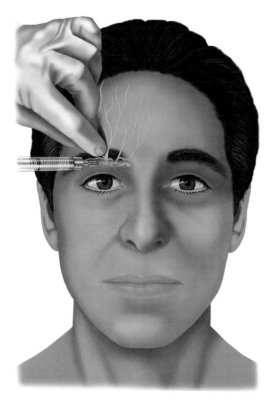

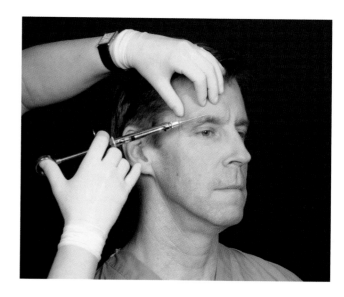

Step 3. Inject anesthetic subcutaneously across the supraorbital ridge.

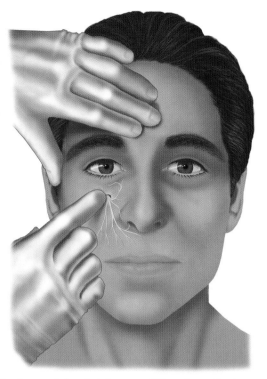
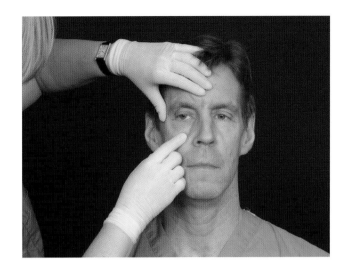

Infraorbital Nerve Block—Extraoral Approach

Step 1. Palpate the infraorbital foramen on the cheek just inferior to the orbital ridge. The foramen will be in a direct line with the pupil when the eye is in the neutral position.

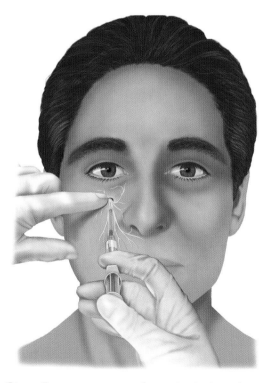
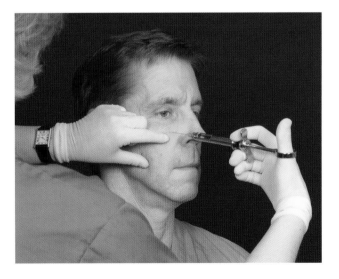

Step 2. Inject 2-3 cc of anesthetic into the area of the infraorbital foramen.

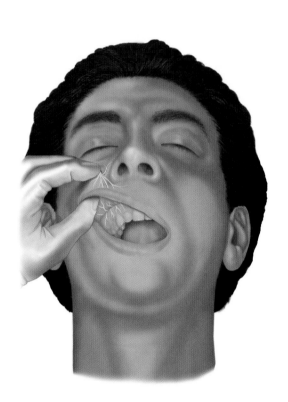 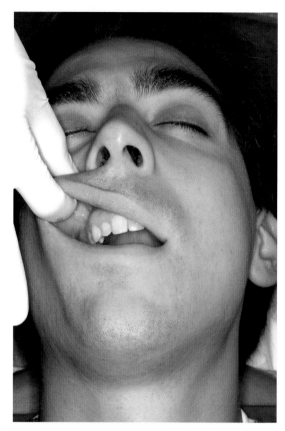

Infraorbital Nerve Block—Intraoral Approach

Step 1. Retract the upper lip and palpate the infraorbital foramen, which can be found just superior to the upper second premolar and in a direct line with the pupil when the eye is in the neutral position.

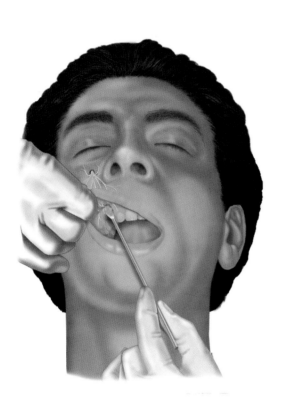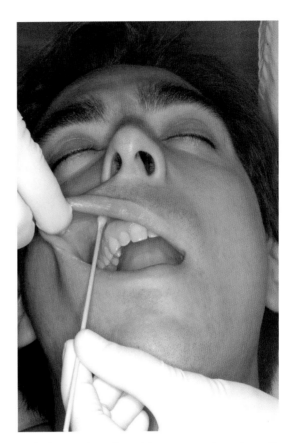

Step 2. Apply topical anesthetic to the mucosa over the intended injection site with a cotton-tipped applicator.

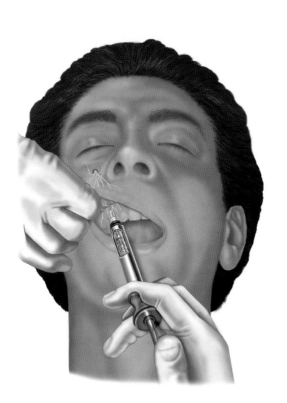
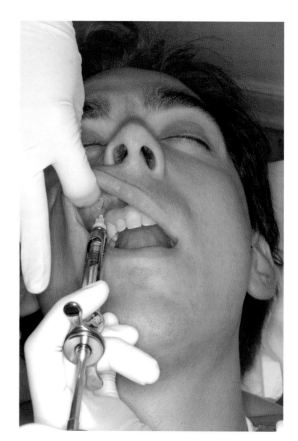

Step 3. Inject 2-3 cc of anesthetic into the area of the infraorbital foramen.

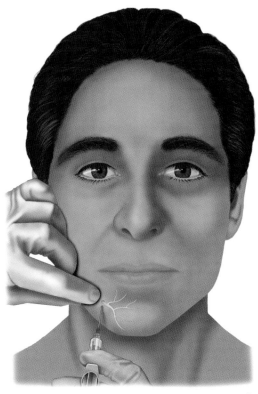 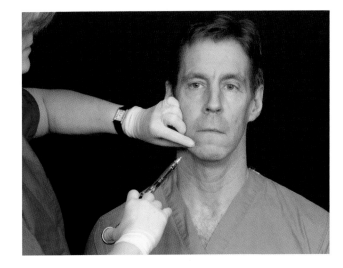

Mental Nerve Block—Extraoral Approach

Step 1. Palpate the mental foramen between the two lower premolar teeth. The foramen will be in a direct line with the pupil when the eye is in the neutral position. Inject 2-3 cc of anesthetic into the area of the mental foramen.

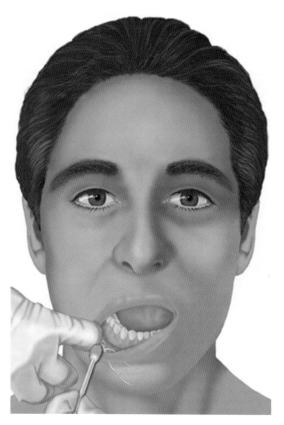

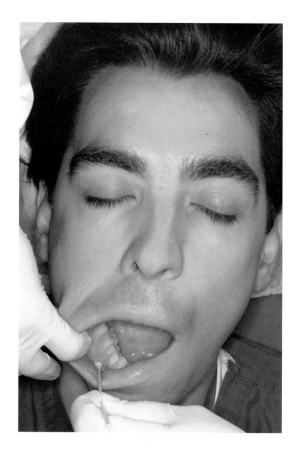

Mental Nerve Block—Intraoral Approach

Step 1. Retract the lower lip. Palpate the mental foramen between the two lower premolar teeth. The foramen will be in a direct line with the pupil when the eye is in the neutral position. Apply topical anesthetic to the mucosa over the intended injection site with a cotton-tipped applicator.

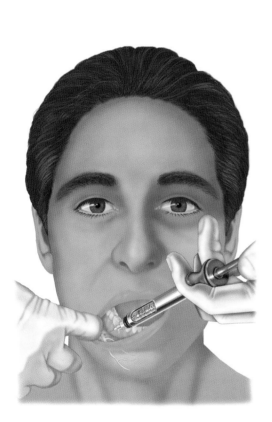

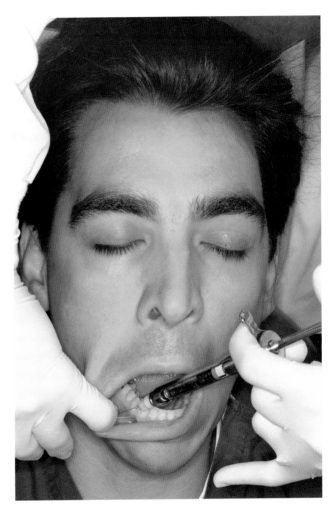

Step 2. Inject 2-3 cc of anesthetic into the mucobuccal fold between the first and second premolars.

Nerve Blocks of the Ear

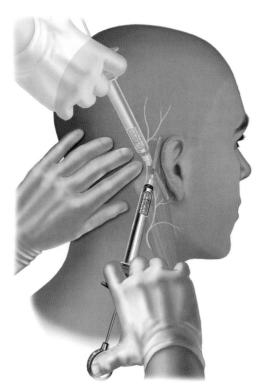

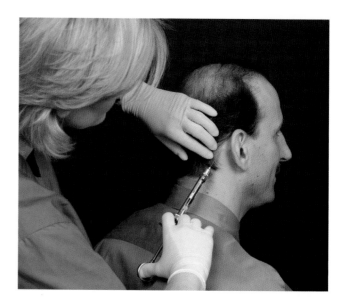

Step 1. Inject anesthetic immediately behind the auricle one half the distance from the inferior to the superior poles of the auricle. Raise a subcutaneous line from the inferior to the superior pole.

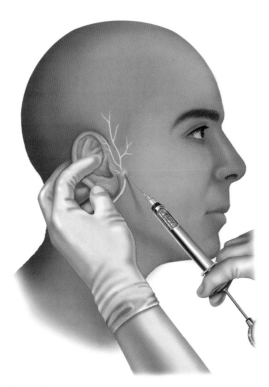

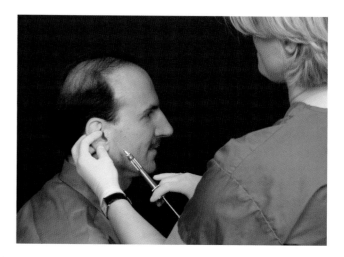

Step 2. Inject 2-3 cc of anesthetic just anterior to the tragus.

Nerve Blocks of the Scalp (Greater and Lesser Occipital Nerves)

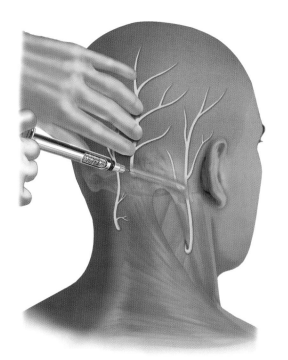 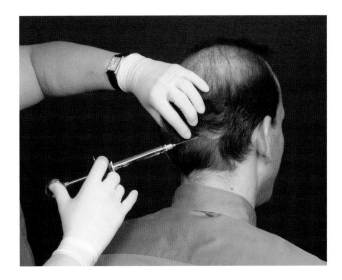

Step 1. Inject 3-5 cc of anesthetic along the nuchal ridge between the external occipital protuberance and the mastoid process.

Nerve Blocks of the Foot

Description:

A nerve block of the foot is a procedure in which anesthetic is injected around a nerve to provide regional anesthesia.

Indications:

- Laceration repair of the foot
- Large area of the foot requiring anesthesia
- Removal of a toenail

Contraindications:

- Injection through an area of infection
- Bleeding diathesis

Complications:

- Bleeding
- Injection of the nerve
- Intravascular injection
- Infection
- Technical failure such as breakage of the needle

Equipment:

A. 25- or 27-gauge needle
B. 5-10 cc syringe
C. 1% or 2% lidocaine solution

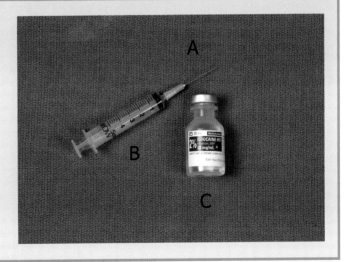

Posterior Tibial Nerve Block

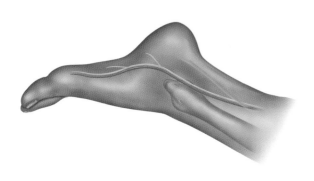
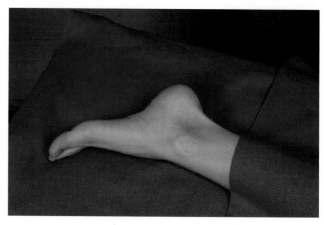

Step 1. Position the patient prone with the foot held in slight dorsiflexion.

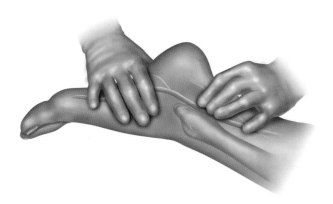
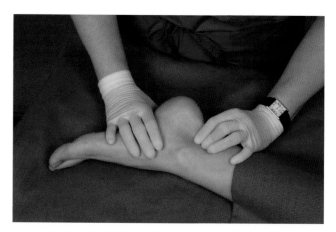

Step 2. Palpate the posterior tibial artery just posterior to the medial malleolus.

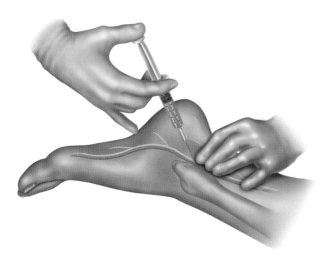 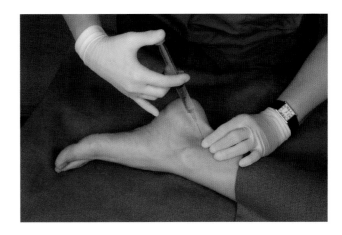

Step 3. Insert the needle just posterior to the artery at the level of the top of the medial malleolus. Aspirate and then inject 3-5 cc of anesthetic.

Sural Nerve Block

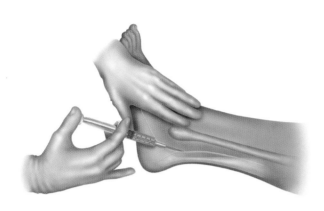 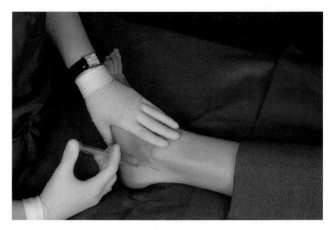

Steps Position the patient supine with the foot held in slight dorsiflexion. Insert the needle lateral to the Achilles tendon and 1 cm superior to the lateral malleolus. Inject a subcutaneous band from just posterior to the lateral malleolus to the Achilles tendon.

Peroneal Nerve Block

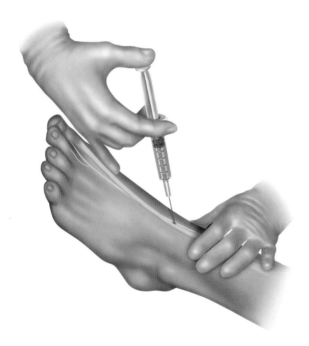 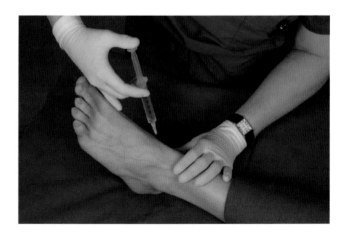

Steps Place the patient supine. Identify the extensor hallucis longus (EHL) tendon by dorsiflexing the great toe. Insert the needle and direct it beneath the EHL tendon at 30 degrees. Inject 3-5 cc of anesthetic. Block the superficial peroneal nerve with a wheal extending anteriorly across the ankle.

Digital Nerve Block of the Toe

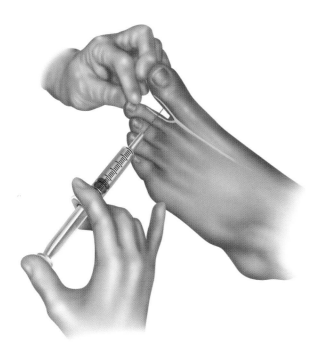

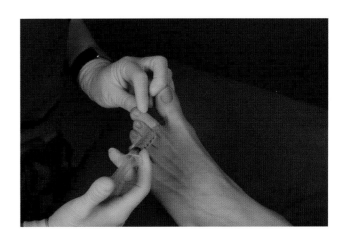

Lateral Approach

Steps Insert the needle at a 90-degree angle to the skin of the toes laterally at the level of the proximal phalanx. Aspirate and then inject 3-5 cc of anesthetic. Repeat on the opposite side of the toe.

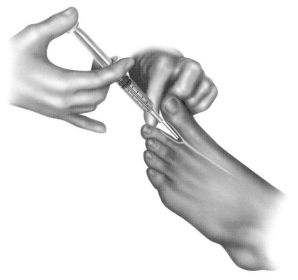

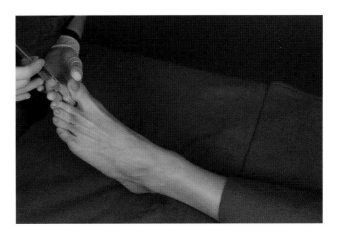

Web Space Approach

Steps Insert the needle into the web space between the toes. Aspirate and then inject 3-5 cc of lidocaine. Repeat on the opposite side of the toe.

Nerve Blocks of the Hand

Description:

A nerve block of the hand is a procedure in which anesthetic is injected around a nerve of the hand to provide regional anesthesia.

Indications:
- Repair of hand laceration
- Removal of a fingernail
- Finger dislocation
- Large surface area of the hand requiring anesthesia

Contraindications:
- Overlying skin infection
- Bleeding diathesis

Complications:
- Bleeding
- Injection of the nerve
- Intravascular injection
- Infection
- Technical failure such as breakage of the needle

Equipment:
A. 25- or 27-gauge needle
B. 5-cc syringe
C. 1% or 2% lidocaine solution

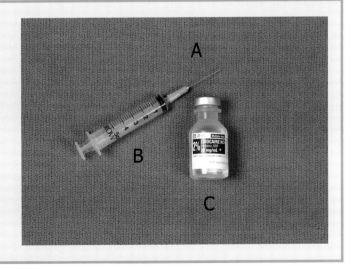

Radial Nerve Block

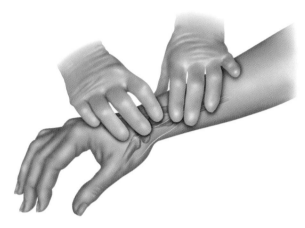

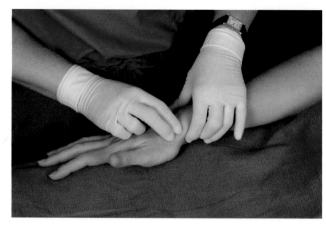

Step 1. Identify the radial artery, radial styloid, and anatomic snuffbox.

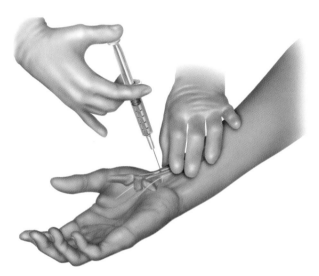

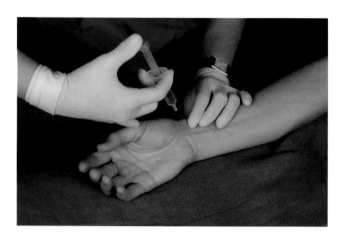

Step 2. At the level of the styloid and just lateral to the radial artery, inject 3 cc of lidocaine.

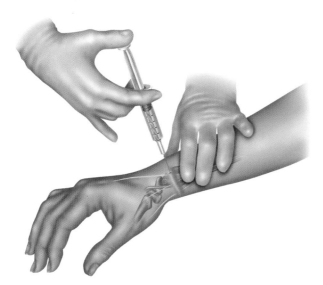 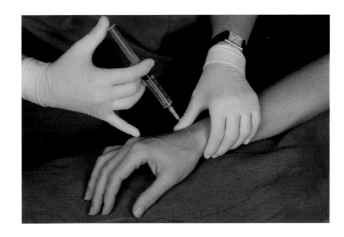

Step 3. Raise a subcutaneous wheal of anesthesia from the deep injection site around the radial surface of the wrist, extending dorsally to the level of the anatomic snuffbox.

Median Nerve Block

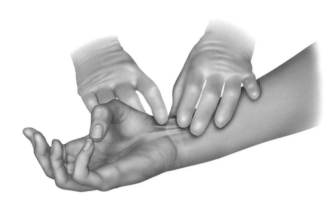

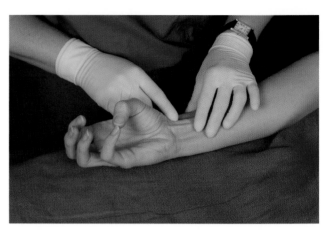

Step 1. Identify the flexor carpi radialis tendon and the palmaris longus tendon by having the patient oppose the thumb and fifth finger while flexing the wrist.

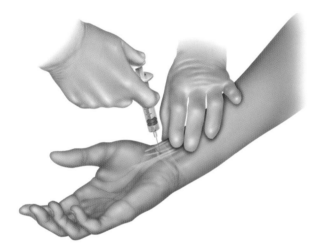

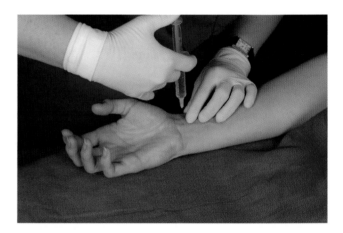

Step 2. At the level of the proximal volar crease, enter with the needle perpendicular to the skin. A pop may be heard as the needle passes through the flexor retinaculum. Once into the deep fascia, inject 5-7 cc of anesthetic.

Ulnar Nerve Block

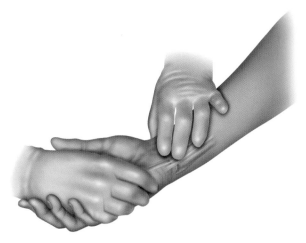

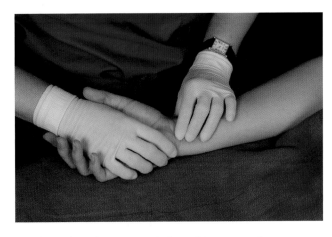

Step 1. Palpate the ulnar artery and the flexor carpi ulnaris tendon. The ulnar nerve is found between these two at the level of the ulnar styloid.

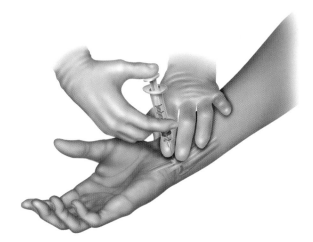

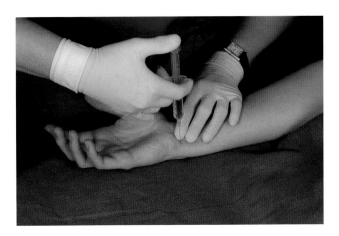

Volar Approach

Steps Insert the needle between the artery and tendon at the proximal palmar crease. Advance the needle until paresthesias are felt, withdraw slightly, and inject 3-5 cc of anesthetic.

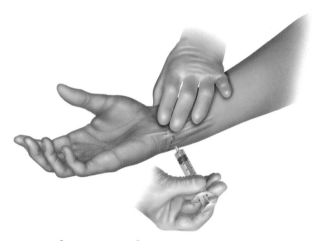 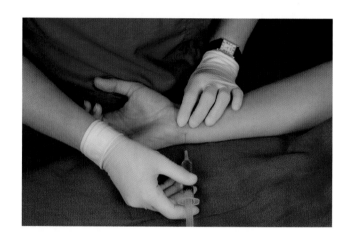

Lateral Approach

Steps Insert the needle under the flexor carpi ulnaris tendon at the proximal palmar crease. Advance the needle until paresthesias are felt, withdraw slightly, and inject 3-5 cc of anesthetic.

Digital Nerve Block of the Finger

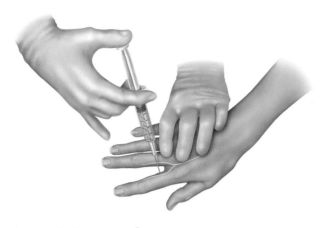

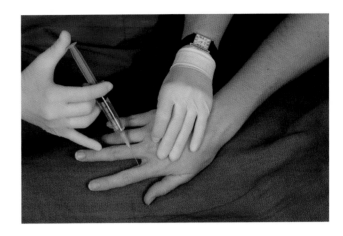

Lateral Approach

Steps Insert the needle at a 90-degree angle to the skin of the finger laterally at the level of the proximal one-third of the proximal phalanx. Aspirate and then inject 3-5 cc of anesthetic. Repeat on the opposite side of the digit.

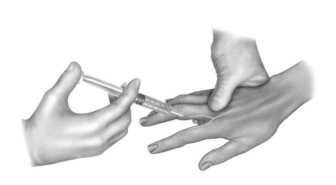

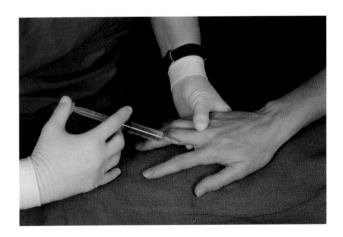

Web Space Approach

Steps Insert the needle into the web space between the fingers. Aspirate and then inject 3-5 cc of anesthetic. Repeat on the opposite side of the digit.

Measurement of Intraocular Pressure: Schiøtz and Tono-Pen Tonometry

Description:

Schiøtz and Tono-Pen tonometry are procedures in which intraocular pressure is measured by the amount of resistance of the globe to indentation by an applied force.

Indications:

- As part of the complete eye examination in the emergency department
- Suspected glaucoma
- Iritis

Contraindications:

Absolute:
- Ruptured globe
- Corneal defects
- Uncooperative patient

Relative:
- Infected eyes (a sterilized cover should be used)

Complications:

- Infection
- Corneal abrasion
- Extrusion of globe contents

Equipment:

- **A.** 0.5% tetracaine anesthetic eye drops
- **B.** Tono-Pen tonometer
- **C.** Latex disposable cover for Tono-Pen tonometer
- **D.** Schiøtz tonometer
- **E.** Weights for Schiøtz tonometer

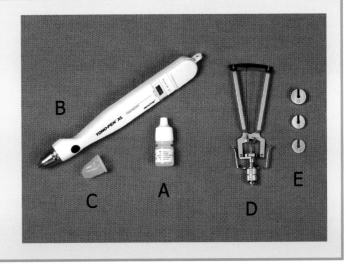

Schiøtz Tonometry

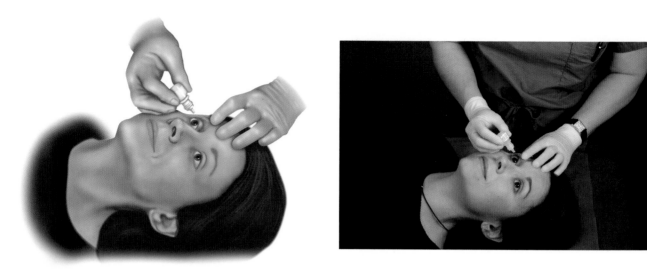

Step 1. Place the patient in the supine position with the face parallel to the stretcher and the ceiling. Instill anesthetic eye drops in the patient's eyes.

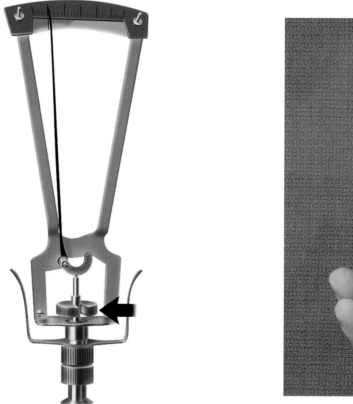

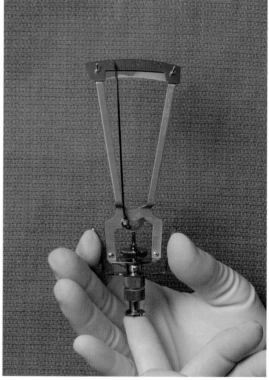

Step 2. Place an appropriate weight on the tonometer, starting with the lowest weight provided.

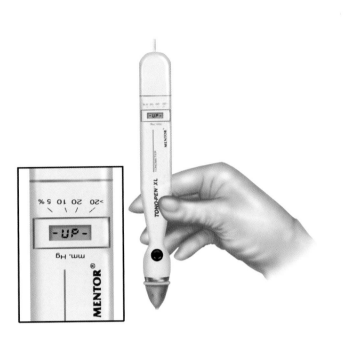

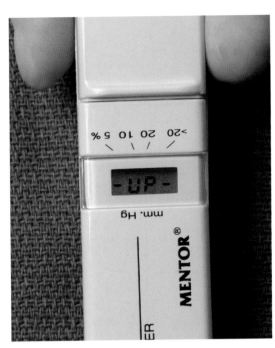

Step 7. Hold the probe with the tip pointing down (for approximately 20 seconds) until a beep sounds and the display "UP" appears.

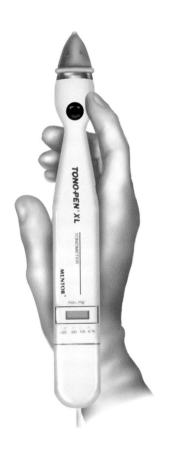

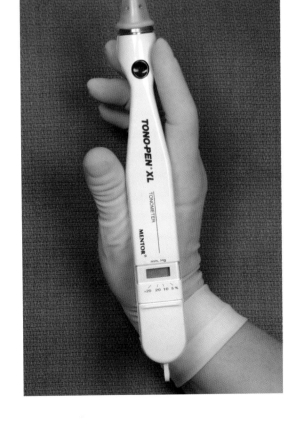

Step 8. Turn the Tono-Pen to the upright position.

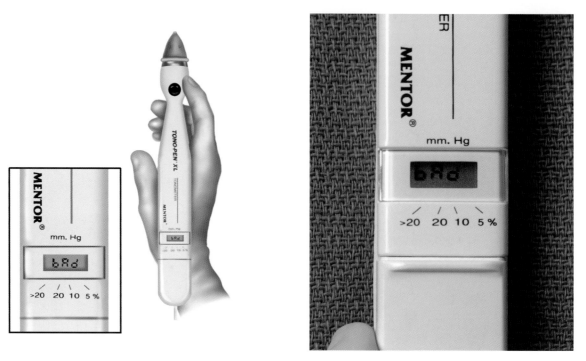

Step 9. Another beep will sound and the display will read "bAd" if the calibration was unsuccessful. If this occurs, repeat the above steps until the calibration is successful.

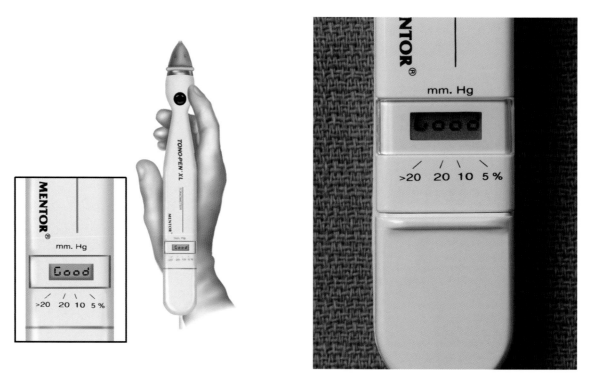

Step 10. The display will read "Good" if the calibration was successful.

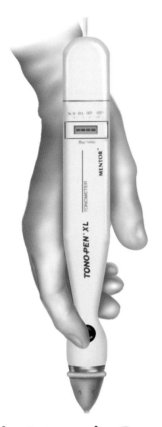

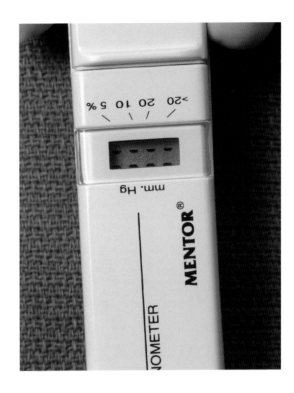

Measure the Intraocular Pressure

Step 11. To measure the intraocular pressure, press and release the activation switch until the display shows "= = = =." A beep will signal this display.

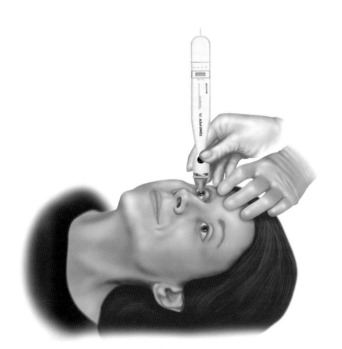

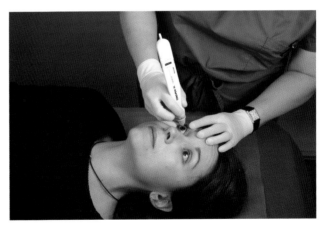

Step 12. Hold the Tono-Pen like a pencil and brace your hand against the patient's cheek to steady the device in case of movement. Lightly touch the pen tip to the cornea four times. A click will sound with each individual measurement.

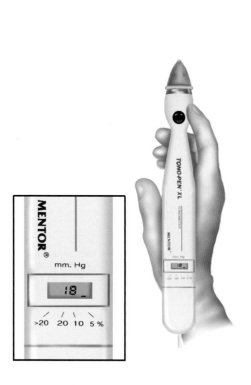

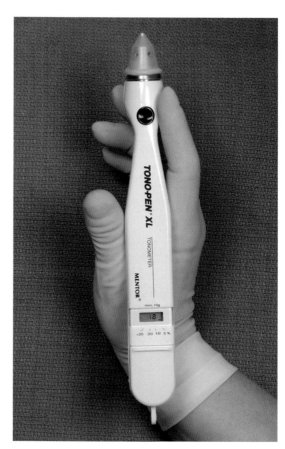

Step 13. After four valid readings, a beep will sound and the average of the measurements will be shown on the display. An associated bar shows the statistical reliability of the measurements. A bar reading greater than 20% indicates that the measurement is unreliable and should be repeated.

Paracentesis

Description:
Paracentesis is a procedure in which a catheter is placed into the peritoneal cavity to remove ascitic fluid for diagnostic and therapeutic purposes.

Indications:
- To determine the etiology of ascites
- To evaluate for bacterial peritonitis
- To remove a large volume of ascitic fluid for therapeutic purposes

Contraindications:
- Overlying skin infection
- Thrombocytopenia
- Severe coagulopathy
- Pregnancy (a relative contraindication)

Complications:
- Infection
- Bleeding
- Abdominal wall hematoma
- Bowel or bladder perforation
- Vascular injury
- Persistent ascitic fluid leak
- Hemodynamic compromise after large-volume paracentesis

Equipment:
A. 1% lidocaine, syringe, and needle for anesthetizing skin
B. 18-gauge angiocatheter
C. 50-cc syringe
D. Intravenous tubing with 3-way stopcock
E. Vacuum container for large-volume paracentesis

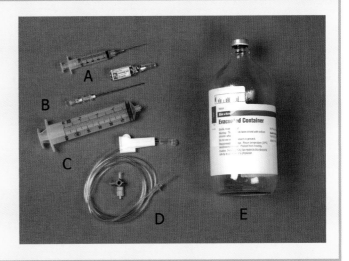

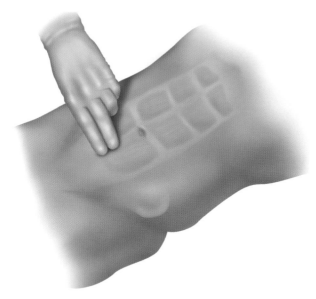

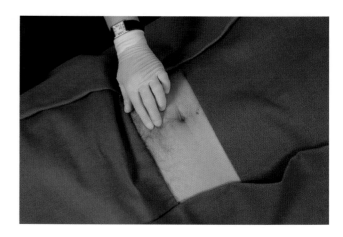

Midline Approach

The site of entry is a few centimeters below the umbilicus.

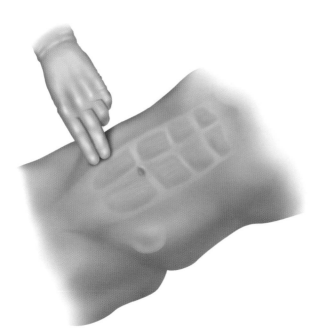

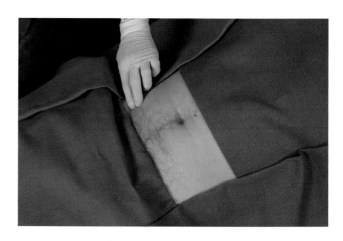

Lateral Approach

The site of entry is just lateral to the rectus muscle in the lower quadrant.

Procedural Steps

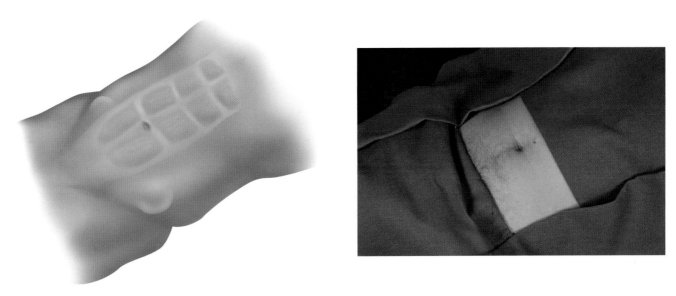

Step 1. Place the patient in a supine, semi-recumbent position.

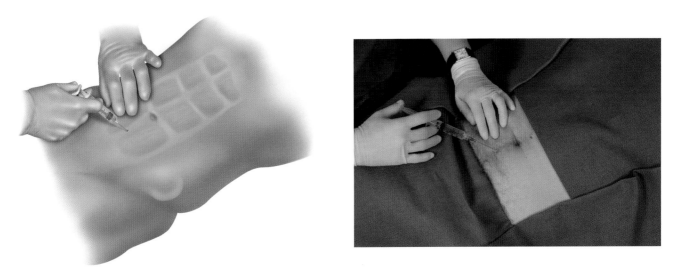

Step 2. Anesthetize the skin at site of entry (see previous page).

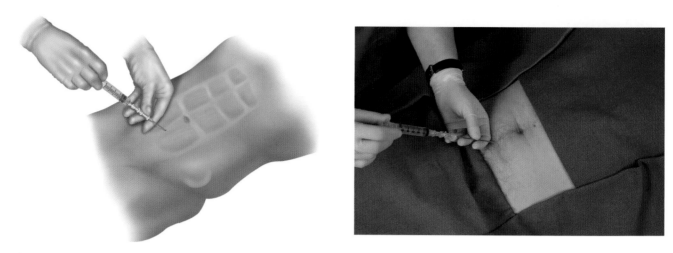

Step 3. Attach the catheter to the syringe and insert at a 70- to 90-degree angle to the skin.

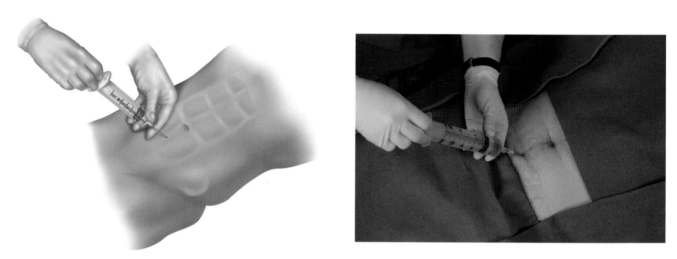

Step 4. Advance the catheter while gently aspirating until ascitic fluid is obtained.

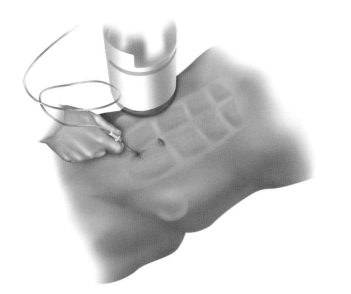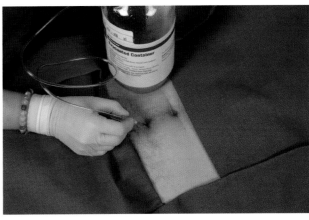

Step 5. For a therapeutic tap, attach one end of the tubing to the catheter and the other by needle to a vacuum container bottle.

Pericardiocentesis

Description:

Pericardiocentesis is a procedure in which a needle is placed in the pericardial space to remove fluid.

Indications:

- Pericardial tamponade, known or suspected
- Cardiac arrest with pulseless electrical activity

Contraindications:

Absolute:
- No evidence of effusion

Relative:
- Coagulopathy

Complications:

- Pneumothorax
- Laceration of the myocardium
- Laceration of the coronary or great vessels
- Air embolism
- New hemopericardium
- Dysrhythmia
- Cardiac arrest
- Infection

Equipment:

A. 18-gauge spinal needle
B. 30-60 cc syringe
C. Flexible guidewire
D. Tissue dilator
E. Pigtail catheter
F. Electrocardiogram (EKG) monitor (not shown)

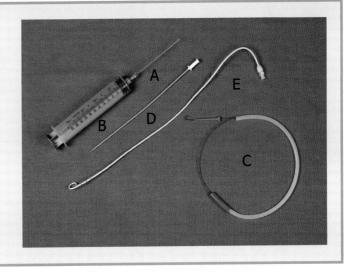

Procedural Steps

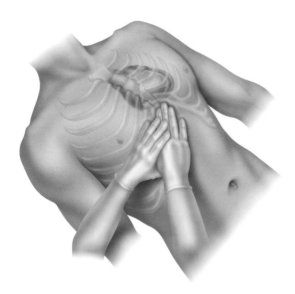

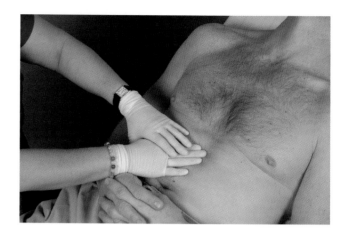

Step 1. Identify the site of insertion between the xiphoid process and the left costal margin.

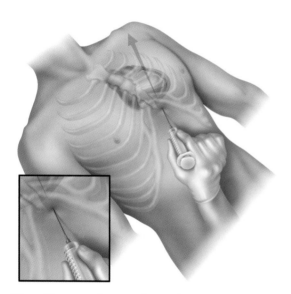

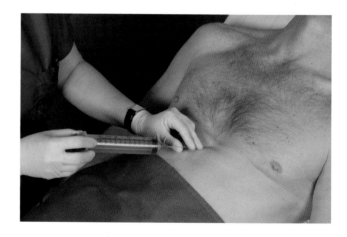

Step 2. Insert the needle in the location shown, at a 30- to 45-degree angle to the skin with the tip directed toward the left shoulder.

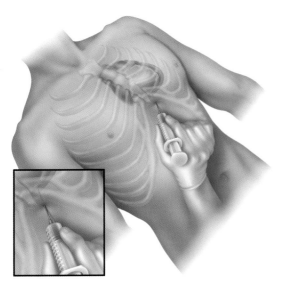

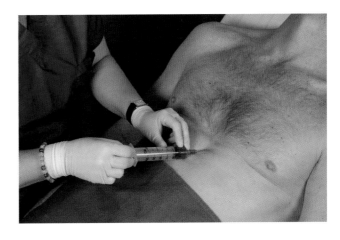

Step 3. Advance the needle until pericardial fluid is obtained. Withdraw pericardial fluid until the desired clinical response is obtained.

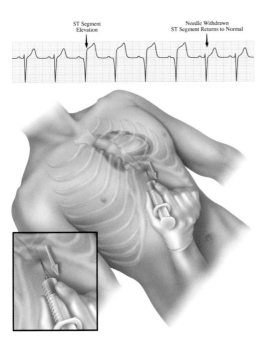

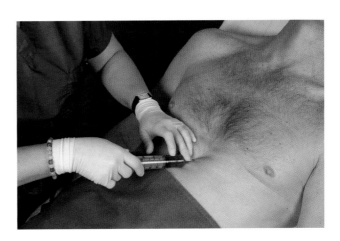

Step 4. If EKG changes are noted, withdraw the needle a small distance.

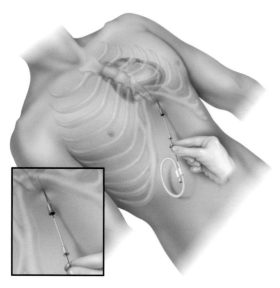

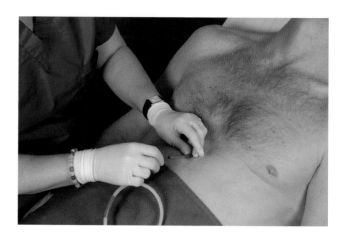

Step 5. Insert a flexible guidewire through the needle.

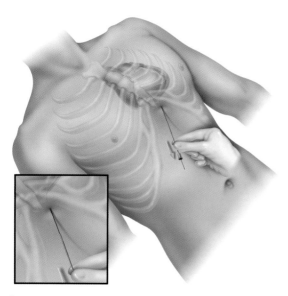

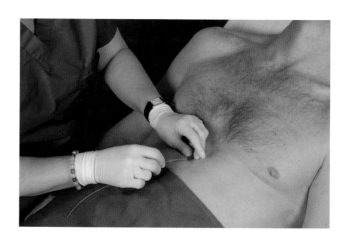

Step 6. Remove the needle.

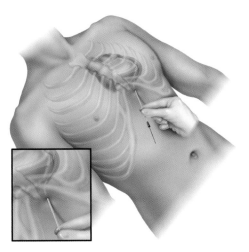

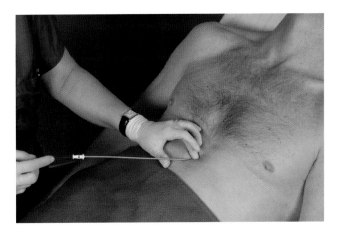

Step 7. Insert a tissue dilator over the guidewire and then remove it, leaving the guidewire in place.

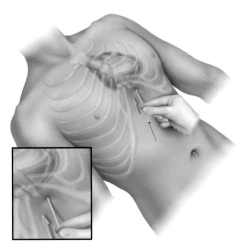

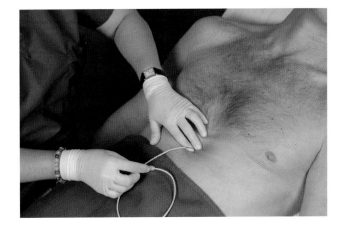

Step 8. Insert a pigtail catheter into the pericardial space.

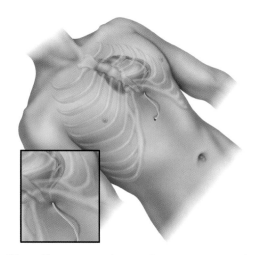 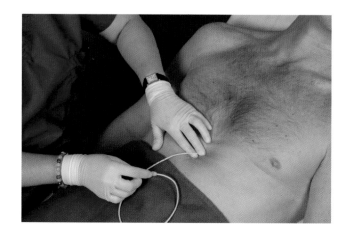

Step 9. Remove the guidewire. Connect the catheter to drainage tubing.

Radial Artery Line Placement

Description:
Radial artery line placement is a procedure in which a catheter is placed into the radial artery.

Indications:
The need for:
- Continuous arterial blood pressure monitoring
- Frequent arterial blood gas sampling

Contraindications:
- Absence of collateral blood flow in the ulnar artery
- Overlying cellulitis
- Major injury to the arm
- Bleeding diathesis

Complications:
- Infection
- Bleeding
- Hematoma
- Thrombosis
- Catheter shear
- Catheter embolization

Equipment:
- **A.** Radial artery catheter (2-inch 20 gauge)
- **B.** Introducer needle, guidewire, and clear tube assembly
- **C.** Plastic skin attachment
- **D.** 4-0 silk for securing the line
- **E.** Pressure tubing
- **F.** Transducer (not shown)

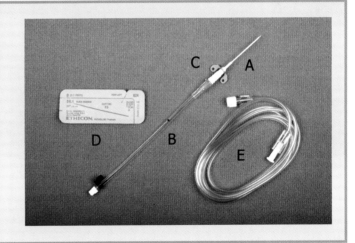

Procedural Steps

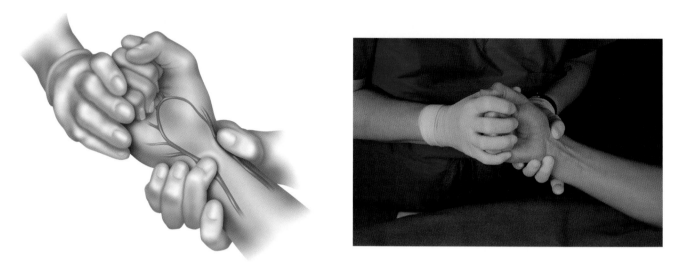

Step 1. Perform the Allen test to assess for patency of the radial and ulnar arteries.

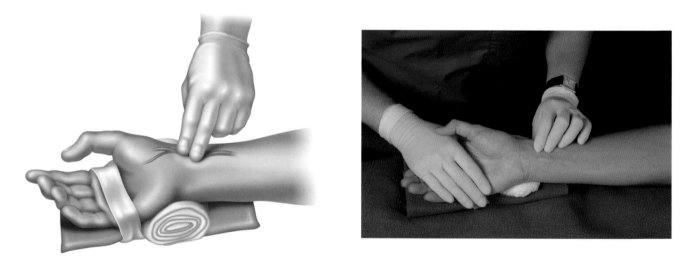

Step 2. Place the wrist palm side up, supported by a rolled-up towel to extend the wrist. Palpate the radial artery.

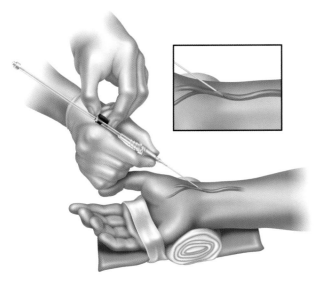
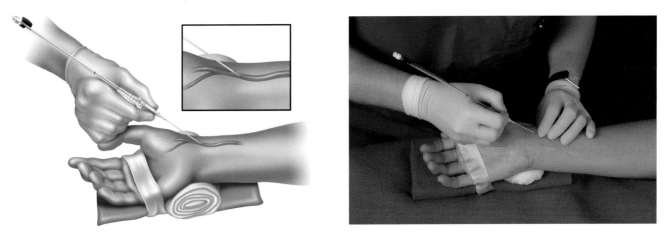

Step 3. Insert the catheter at a 45-degree angle cephalad and advance until arterial blood is seen.

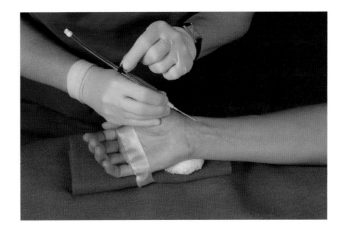

Step 4. Advance the guidewire into the artery.

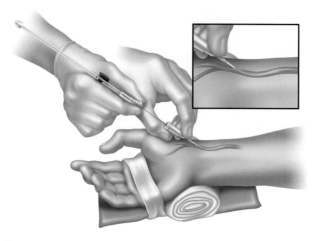 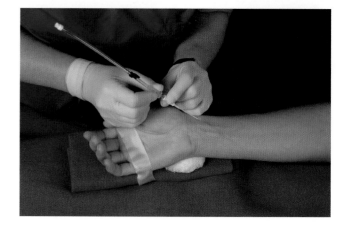

Step 5. Advance the catheter over the guidewire.

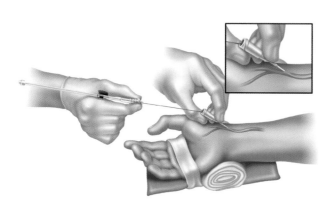 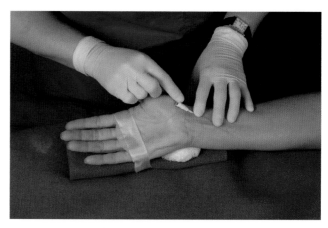

Step 6. Remove the introducer needle, guidewire, and clear tube assembly. Confirm pulsatile flow.

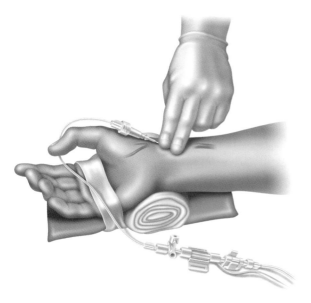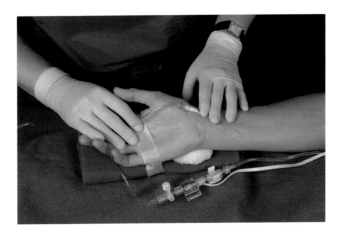

Step 7. Attach a stopcock and pressure tubing. Flush the catheter and tubing.

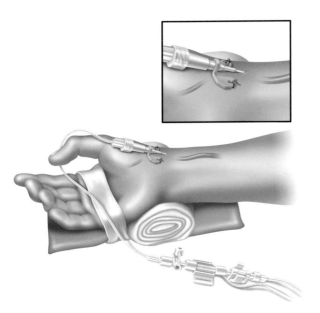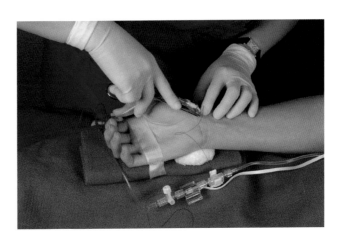

Step 8. Secure the catheter to the skin with suture and plastic skin attachment.

Raney Clip Application

Description:
Raney clip application is a procedure in which clips are placed on the wound edges of a scalp laceration for control of bleeding.

Indication:
- Vigorously bleeding scalp wounds

Contraindication:
- None

Complications:
- Persistent bleeding of the scalp
- Infection

Equipment:
A. Raney clip applicator
B. Raney clips

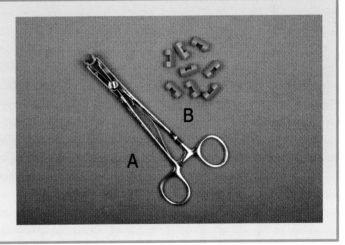

Procedural Steps

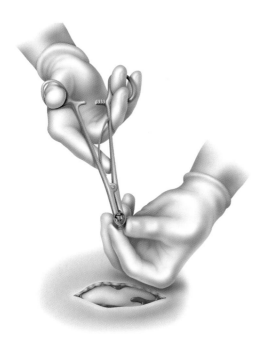

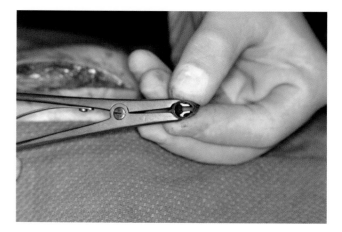

Step 1. Load the clip onto the applicator.

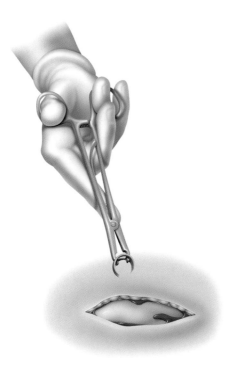

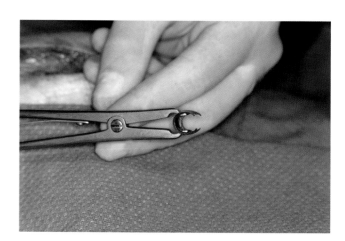

Step 2. Lock the handles of the applicator to open the clip.

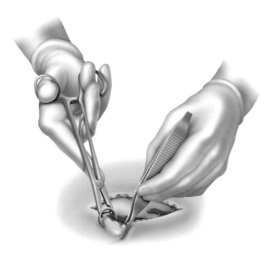

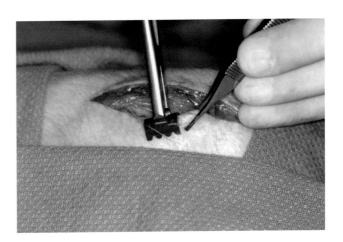

Step 3. Slide the clip onto the wound edge.

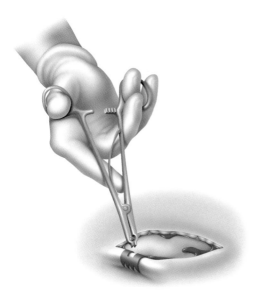

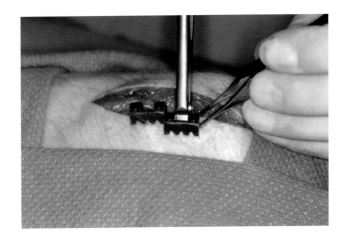

Step 4. Release the clip by unlocking the applicator.

Suprapubic Bladder Aspiration

Description:
Suprapubic bladder aspiration is a procedure in which a needle is inserted through the abdominal wall into the bladder to obtain a urine specimen.

Indications:
To obtain urine:
- In a young child when otherwise not obtainable
- In traumatic urethral injury
- In the presence of phimosis
- To relieve acute urinary retention when it is impossible to pass a urethral catheter

Contraindications:
- Lower abdominal scars from previous surgery
- Small or non-palpable bladder

Complications:
- Gross hematuria
- Bowel perforation
- Large vessel puncture
- Abdominal wall hematoma
- Abdominal wall abscess
- Leakage around the catheter
- Urinoma

Equipment:
- **A.** 1% lidocaine solution with needle and syringe for anesthetizing skin
- **B.** 19-gauge needle
- **C.** 10-cc syringe
- **D.** Sterile specimen container

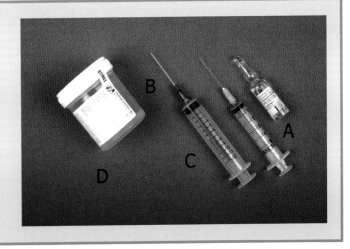

Procedural Steps

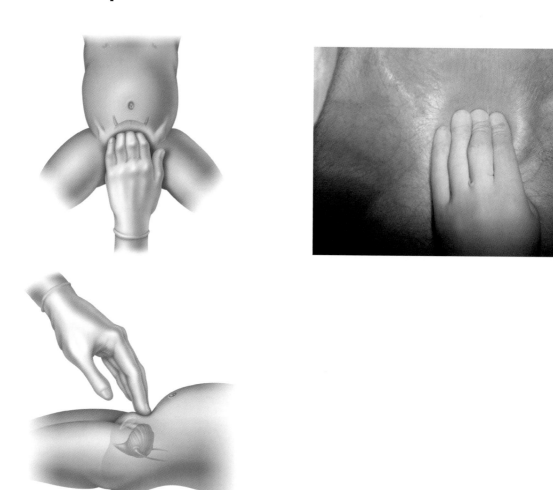

Step 1. Identify a point 1-2 cm above the symphysis pubis. Locate and palpate the bladder.

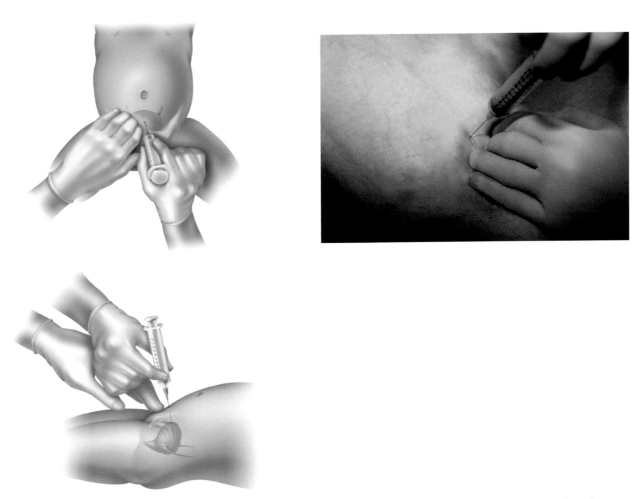

Step 2. Insert a 19-gauge needle at a 10- to 20-degree angle, in the cephalad direction in children and in the caudad direction in adults.

Thoracentesis

Description:

Thoracentesis is a procedure in which a catheter is placed into the pleural space to obtain fluid for diagnostic or therapeutic purposes.

Indications:
- Diagnostic evaluation of pleural effusions
- Drainage of large pleural effusions for therapeutic reasons

Contraindications:
- Ruptured diaphragm
- Chest wall infection
- Loculated effusions
- Pleural adhesions
- Bleeding diathesis

Complications:
- Pneumothorax
- Hemothorax
- Laceration of the lung
- Injury to the diaphragm
- Transient hypoxia
- Re-expansion pulmonary edema
- Infection
- Cough
- Shearing of the catheter

Equipment:
- **A.** 1% lidocaine solution, syringe, and needle for anesthetizing the skin
- **B.** 16- or 20-gauge angiocatheter with 10-cc syringe for aspirating
- **C.** 60-cc syringe
- **D.** Sterile IV tubing with three-way stopcock
- **E.** Vacuum collection bottle
- **F.** Sterile specimen containers

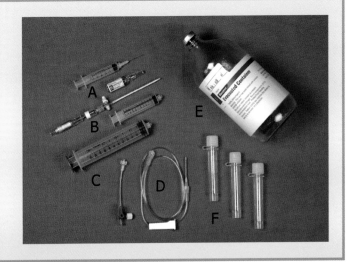

Procedural Steps

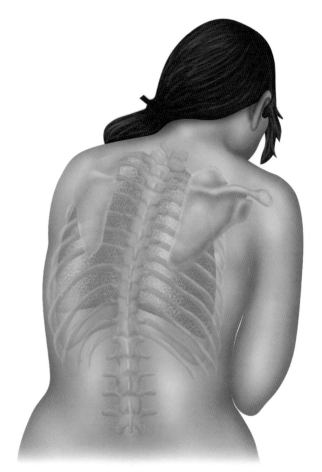

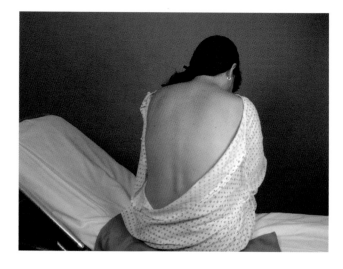

Step 1. Place the patient in a sitting position leaning over a stand.

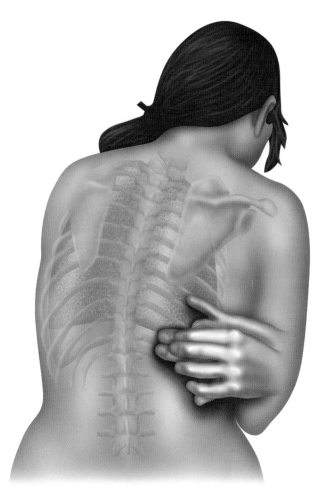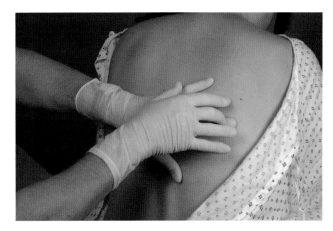

Step 2. Percuss the patient's back to locate the level of the effusion.

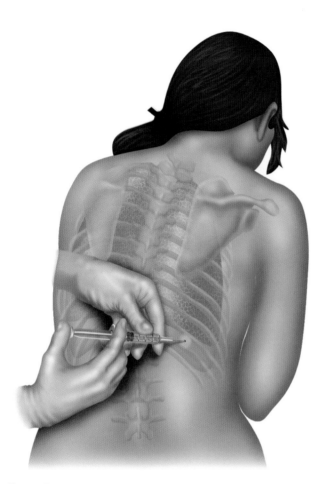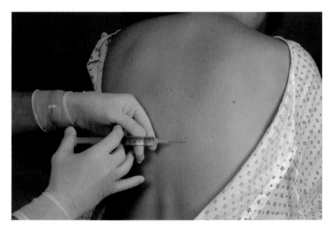

Step 3. Anesthetize the skin over the insertion site with 1% lidocaine.

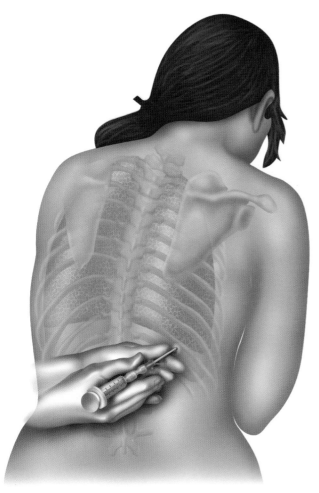

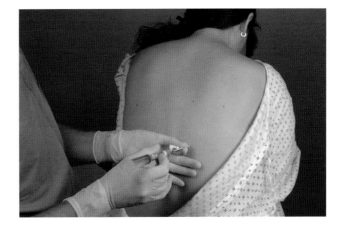

Step 4. Attach the catheter and stopcock to a syringe. Insert the catheter at the indicated rib interspace at the midscapular or posterior axillary line.

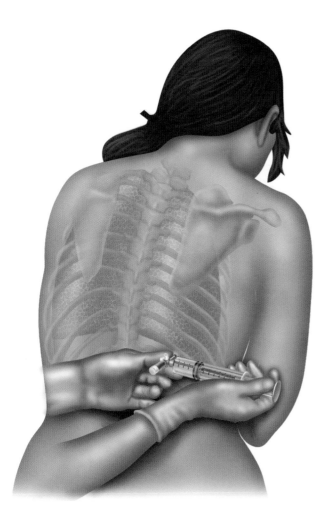

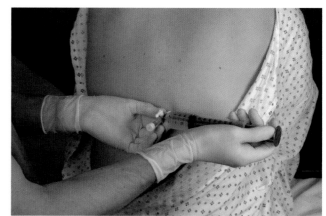

Step 5. Advance the catheter into the pleural space and aspirate for fluid.

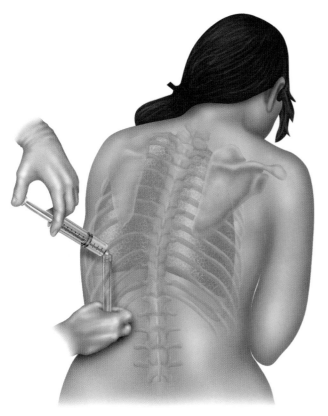 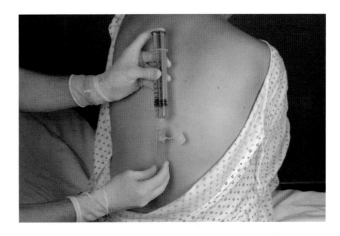

Step 6. For a diagnostic tap, remove sufficient fluid to send to the laboratory for analysis, and remove the catheter.

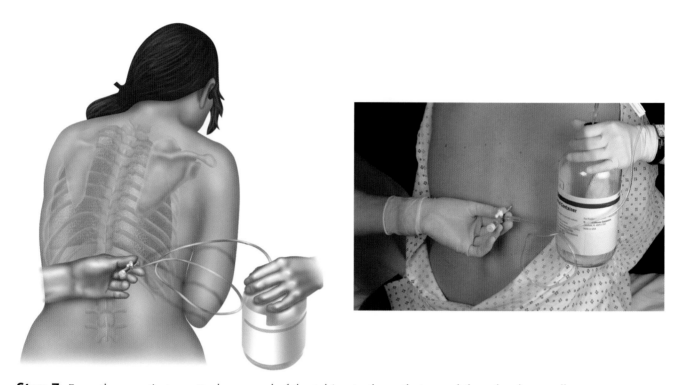

Step 7. For a therapeutic tap, attach one end of the tubing to the catheter and the other by needle to a vacuum collection bottle. Remove the catheter.

Thoracotomy

Description:
Thoracotomy is a procedure in which the chest is opened to release cardiac tamponade, control hemorrhage from the heart, perform direct cardiac massage, cross-clamp the aorta, and/or internally defibrillate the heart.

Indications:
- Penetrating trauma with loss of vital signs during transport or in the emergency department
- Blunt trauma with loss of vital signs in the emergency department

Contraindications:
- Clinically stable patient
- Obvious signs of death (e.g., rigor mortis or decapitation)
- Blunt trauma resulting in cardiopulmonary arrest in the field

Complications:
- Laceration of the lung
- Laceration of the heart or coronary vessels
- Laceration of the internal mammary arteries
- Avulsion of the lumbar veins
- Injuries to the intercostal neurovascular bundle
- Survival of the patient in a vegetative state

Equipment:
A. Scalpel—No. 10 or 22 blade
B. Curved scissors
C. Straight scissors
D. Rib retractor
E. Toothed forceps
F. Vascular clamp
G. Liebsche knife or sternal osteotome with hammer
H. Long needle holder
I. No. 0-0 silk suture

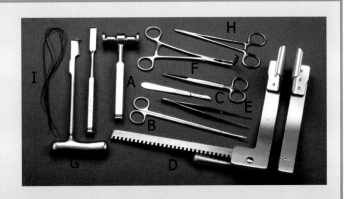

Procedural Steps

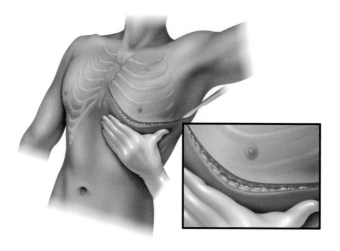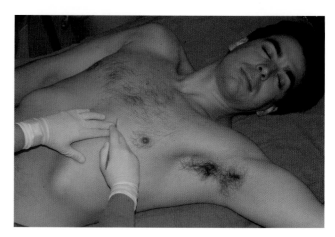

Step 1. Make a left anterolateral incision from sternum to midaxillary line at the fourth to fifth intercostal space.

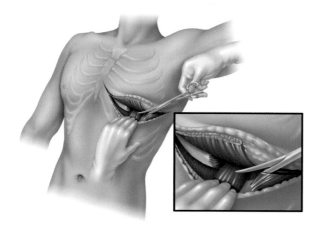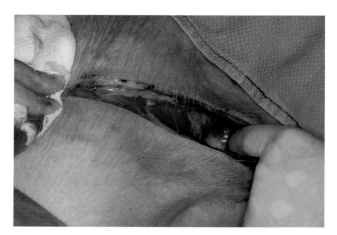

Step 2. Cut through the chest wall muscles with curved scissors.

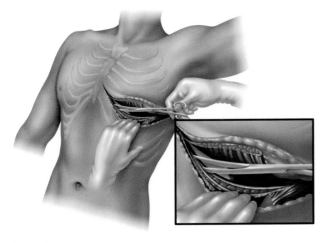

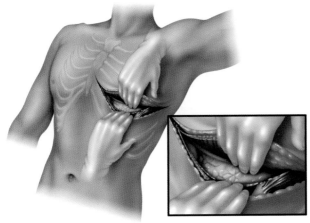

Step 3. Cut the parietal pleura.

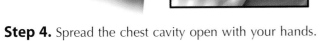

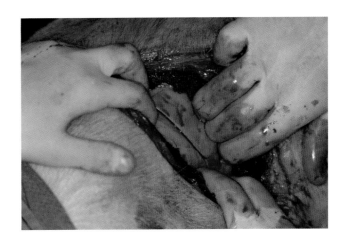

Step 4. Spread the chest cavity open with your hands.

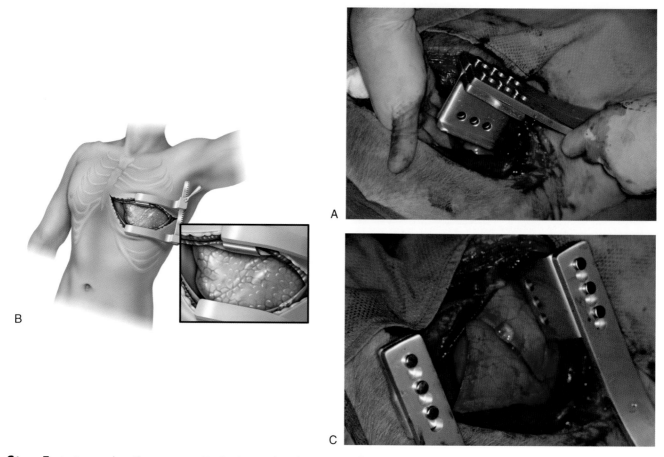

Step 5. A, Insert the rib retractor. **B, C,** Open the chest cavity by turning the handles of the rib retractor. The Liebsche knife or sternal osteotome with hammer may be used to extend the incision to the right side of the chest if necessary.

154

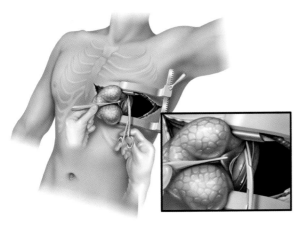 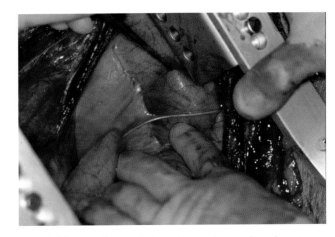

Step 6. Open the pericardial sac with scissors. The incision should be made medial and anterior to the phrenic nerve.

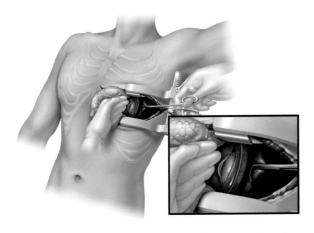 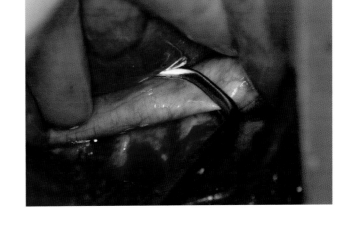

Step 7. Cross-clamp the aorta with a vascular clamp.

Tube Thoracostomy

Description:
Tube thoracostomy is a procedure in which a tube is placed into the pleural cavity to drain abnormal collections of air or fluid.

Indications:
- Pneumothorax
- Hemothorax
- Hemopneumothorax
- Empyema
- Chylothorax
- Recurrent pleural effusion

Contraindications:
- Multiple adhesions
- Pulmonary blebs
- Immediate need for open thoracotomy
- Bleeding diathesis
- Overlying skin infection

Complications:
- Lung laceration
- Laceration of intercostal vessels and nerves
- Laceration of the long thoracic nerve
- Puncture of solid organs
- Re-expansion pulmonary edema
- Infection
- Bleeding
- Mechanical problems, such as failure to drain or kinking of tube

Equipment:

A. 1% lidocaine, needle and syringe
for anesthetizing the skin

B. Scalpel, No. 10 blade

C. Large Kelly clamp

D. Straight scissors

E. Chest tube

F. 1-0 silk suture

G. Needle holder

H. Vaseline gauze

I. Drain sponges

J. Elastic tape

K. Drainage system

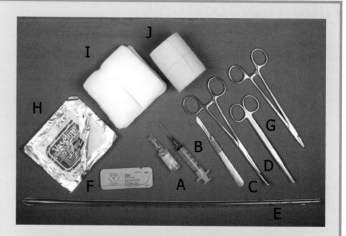

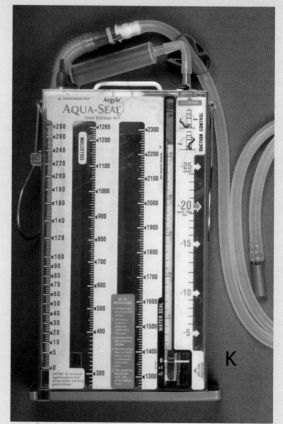

Procedural Steps

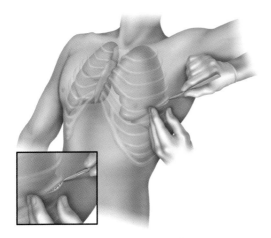

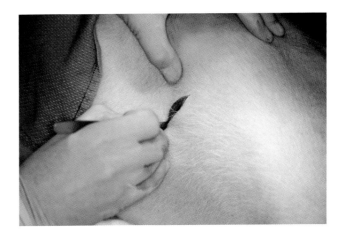

Step 1. Anesthetize the skin. Make an incision over the rib below the fourth to fifth intercostal space at the midaxillary line.

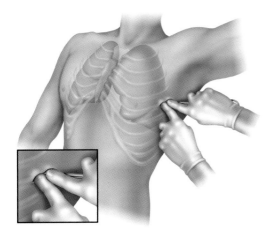

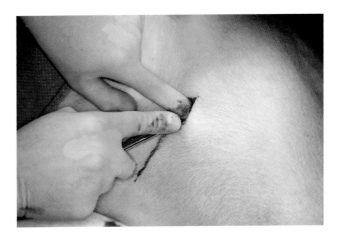

Step 2. Bluntly dissect the subcutaneous tissues overlying the intercostal muscles.

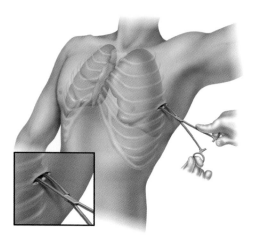
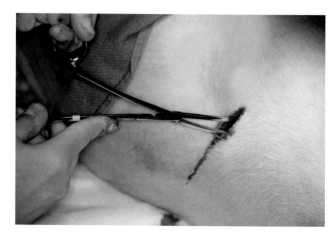

Step 3. Push through the muscles and pleura with a clamp.

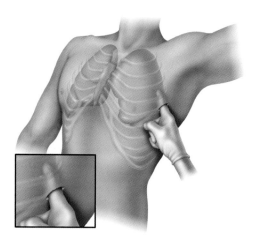
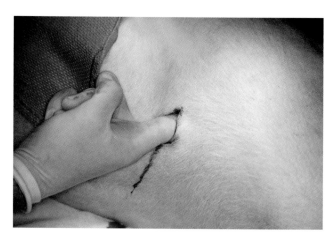

Step 4. Insert a gloved finger to check for pleural adhesions.

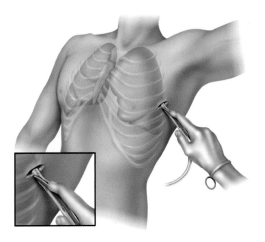
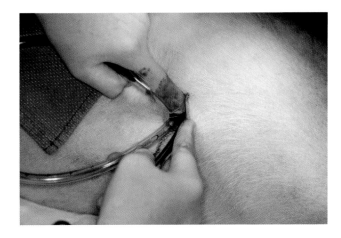

Step 5. Grasp the tube with the clamp and insert it into the pleural space.

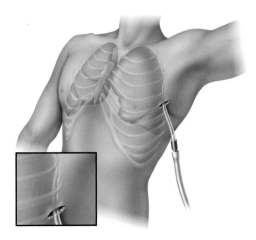
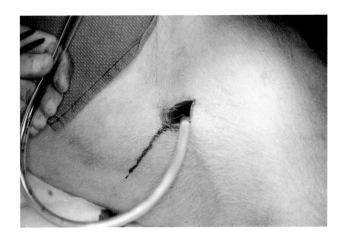

Step 6. Guide the tube superiorly and posteriorly until all side holes are inside the chest. Attach to drainage system.

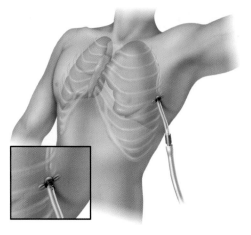
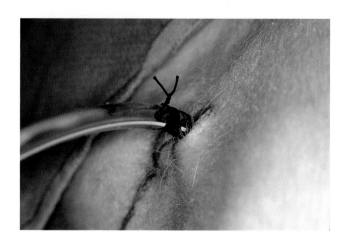

Step 7. Secure the tube with suture.

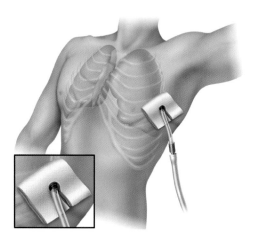
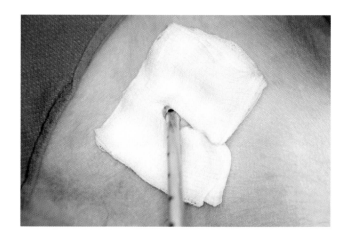

Step 8. Cover with drain sponges and a compressive bandage.

Venous Cutdown: Saphenous and Femoral Vein Approaches

Description:
Venous cutdown is a procedure in which venous access may be rapidly obtained by cutting through skin and soft tissues, exposing a peripheral vein and cannulating it.

Indications:
As an alternative to venipuncture in critically ill patients in need of vascular access and in whom venipuncture may be difficult. Examples include:
- Shock
- Small children
- Sclerosed veins of intravenous drug abusers

Contraindications:
Absolute:
- When less invasive options exist for venous access

Relative:
- Bleeding diathesis
- Overlying skin infection
- Immunocompromise
- Extremity injuries proximal to the site

Complications:
- Transection of the vein
- Transection of an artery
- Bleeding
- Hematoma
- Phlebitis
- Thrombus formation
- Injury to surrounding structures

Equipment:
A. Scalpel—No. 11 blade
B. Curved hemostat
C. No. 0-0 silk suture
D. Iris scissors
E. Plastic venous dilator
F. Large-bore intravenous catheter
G. Intravenous tubing
H. Tape for securing catheter

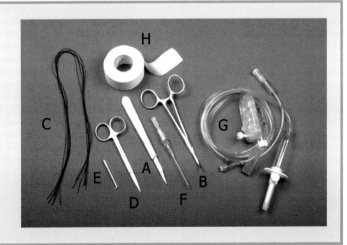

Procedural Steps

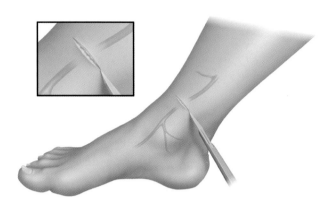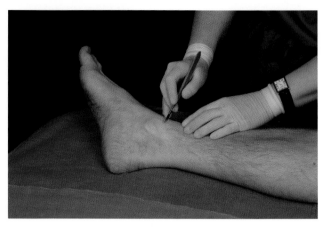

Step 1A. (Saphenous vein approach): The saphenous vein at the ankle can be found approximately 1 cm anterior to the medial malleolus. Make a skin incision perpendicular to the course of the vein.

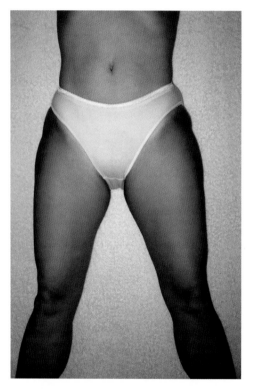

Step 1B. (Femoral vein approach): The femoral vein at the thigh can be found by palpating the femoral artery pulse just inferior to the inguinal ligament, midway between the anterior superior iliac spine and the pubic tubercle. The femoral vein will be found just medial to the artery. Once the vein is located, the procedure shown here for the saphenous vein is essentially the same for the femoral vein.

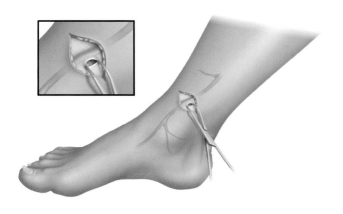
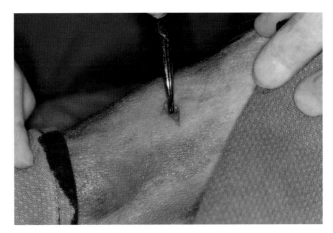

Step 2. Bluntly dissect, isolate, and mobilize the vein.

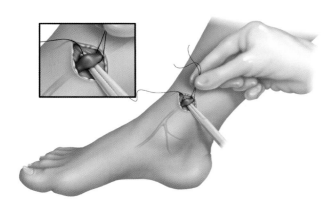
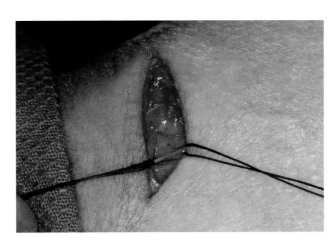

Step 3. Pass silk ties under the vein proximal and distal to the proposed cannulation site.

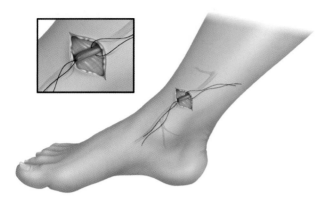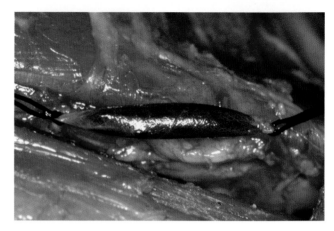

Step 4. Tie the distal suture only.

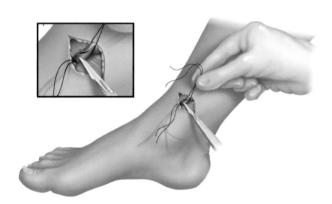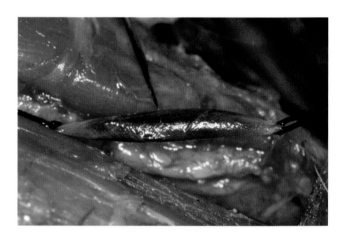

Step 5. Incise the vein while retracting the proximal ligature.

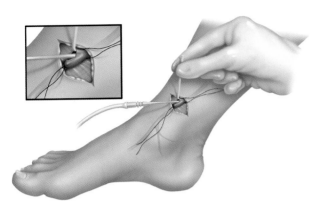 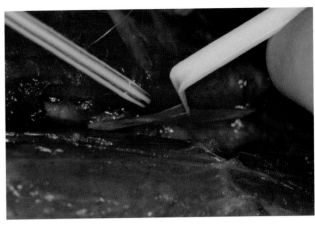

Step 6. Using the plastic venous dilator to lift the flap, advance the catheter into the vein. Attach intravenous tubing to the catheter.

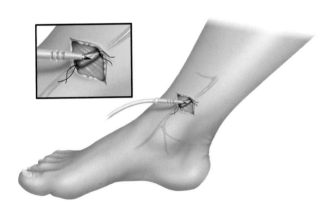 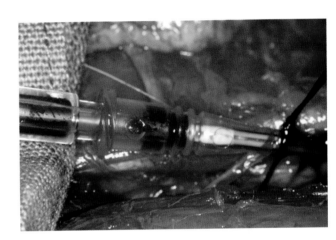

Step 7. Tie the proximal silk suture around the vein and catheter.

Wound Care Procedures

Description:
Wound repair techniques are procedures in which the edges of a wound are brought together to allow more rapid healing with minimal scar formation.

Indication:
- Laceration repair

Contraindications:
Consider these factors in assessing the risk of complications and weigh these risks against the benefits of the procedure.
- Infection
- Wound location
- Contamination (especially animal or human bites)
- Delay in seeking care (especially a wound more than 12 hours old)

Complication:
- Infection
- Bleeding
- Hematoma formation
- Wound dehiscence
- Scar formation

Equipment: Suturing
A. 1% lidocaine, 27-gauge needle, and syringe for anesthetizing skin
B. Wound irrigation device and normal saline
C. Suture scissors
D. Toothed forceps
E. Needle holder
F. Suture with curved needle
G. Gauze dressings

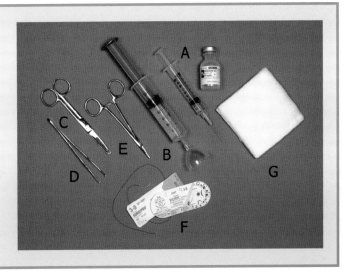

Equipment: Staple Application and Removal

A. Staple applicator
B. Staples
C. Staple remover

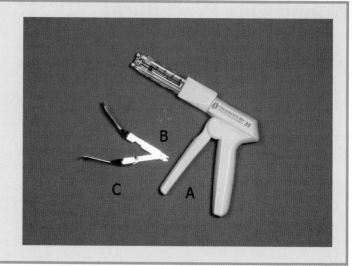

Equipment: Wound Closure Tape Application

A. Wound closure tape strips
B. Adhesive solution such as benzoin
C. Scissors

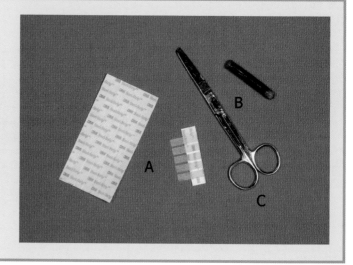

Preparing the Skin for Wound Repair

To prepare the skin, the wound is anesthetized, cleaned, and debrided prior to repair of the laceration.

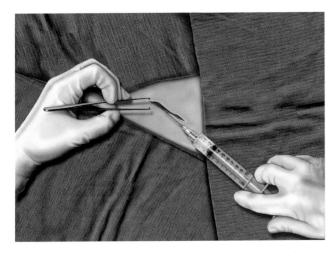 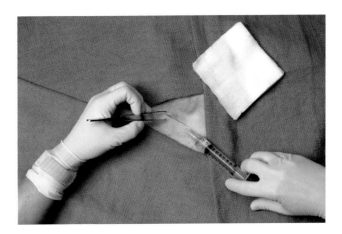

Step 1. After performing a complete neurovascular examination, anesthetize the wound. Drape the wound with sterile towels.

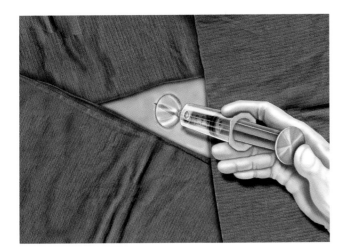 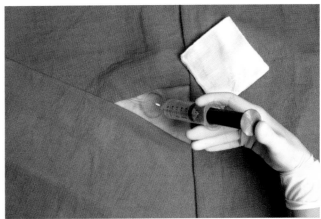

Step 2. Cleanse, irrigate, and debride the wound if necessary. Explore the wound for injury to surrounding structures and for foreign bodies.

Instrument Tie

In the instrument tie technique, a needle holder is used to tie a square knot in the skin. A square knot is one in which the two halves of the knot are mirror images.

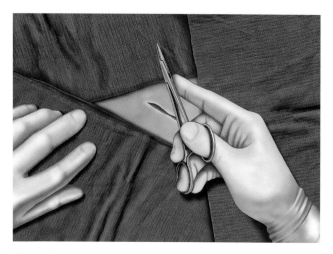

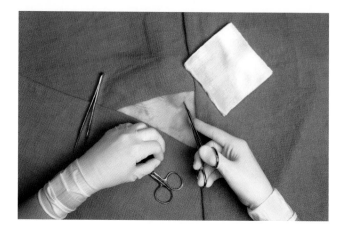

Step 1. Using the dominant hand, grasp the needle holder with the thumb through one of the instrument's finger rings and with the ring finger through the other finger ring.

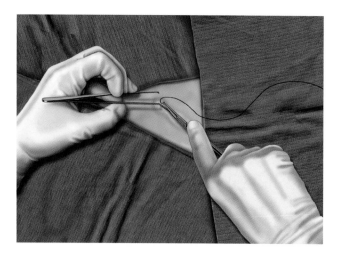

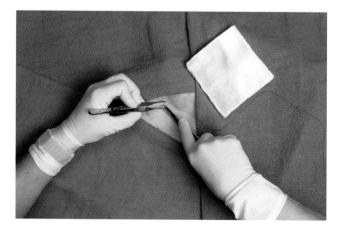

Step 2. Grasp the curved needle of the suture with the needle holder at approximately one-third of the distance from the attachment of the suture to the tip of the needle. Hold the toothed forceps in the non-dominant hand and use them to evert the edges of the wound. Forceps should not be clamped on the outer portion of the skin.

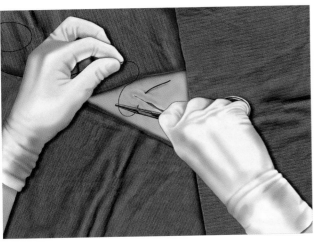
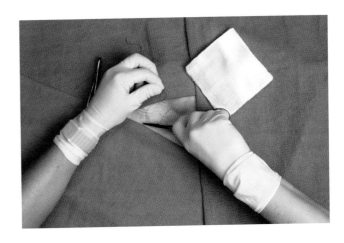

Step 3. Place a suture as described in the following sections. Grasp the end of the suture that has the needle attached to it. Pull the suture through the skin until a short length remains.

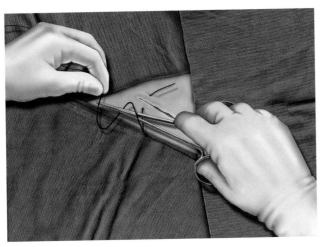
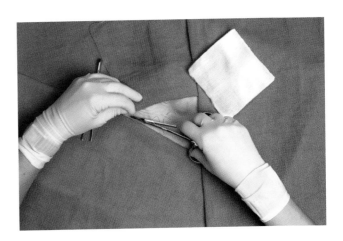

Step 4. Wrap the suture around the needle holder twice for the first throw.

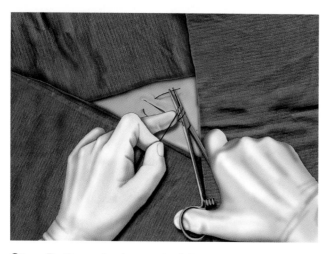 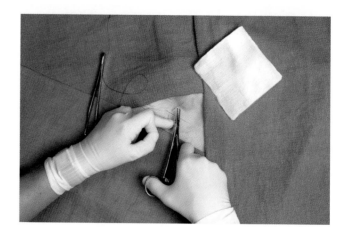

Step 5. Grasp the free end of the suture with the needle holder.

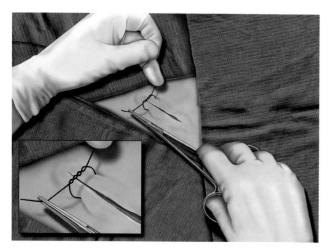 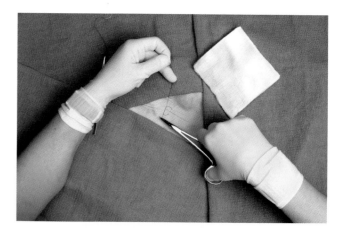

Step 6. Pull the free end of the suture through the two loops that were previously wrapped around the needle holder. Tighten the first half of the knot, bringing it close to the skin surface.

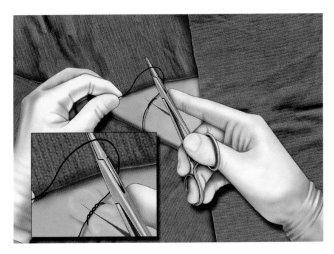
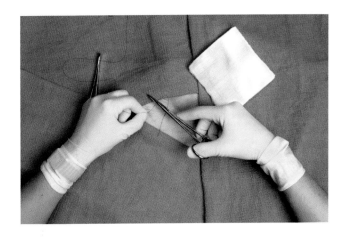

Step 7. For the second half of the knot, wrap the long end of the suture around the needle holder only once in the opposite direction from the original loops.

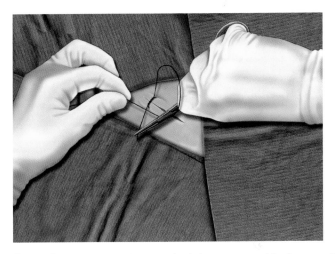
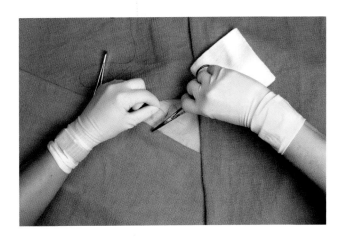

Step 8. Grasp the short end of the suture with the needle holder.

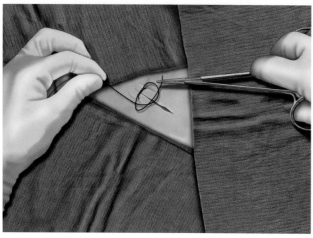
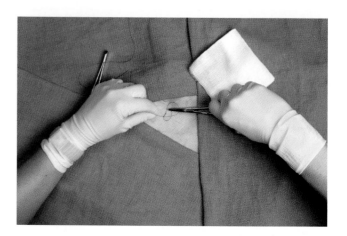

Step 9. Pull the short end through the loop.

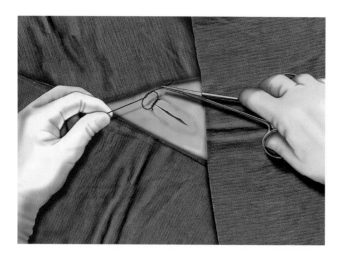
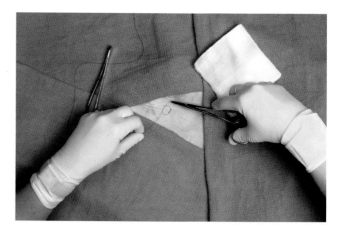

Step 10. Pull down the second half and complete the square knot.

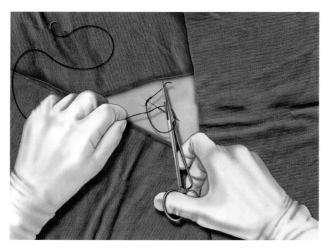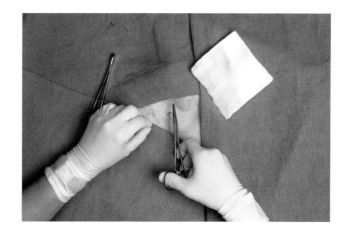

Step 11. Additional throws (most commonly three) may be tied on top of the first knot in alternating directions.

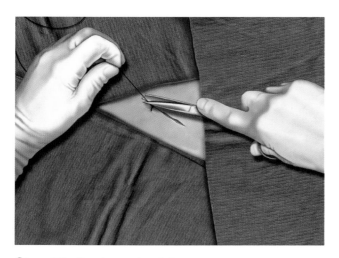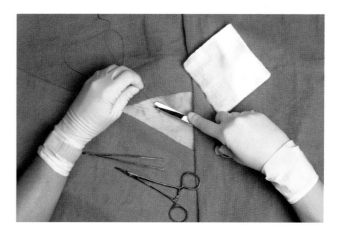

Step 12. Cut the ends of the suture.

Simple Interrupted Suture

In the simple interrupted suture technique, single sutures are placed and tied separately along the wound edge.

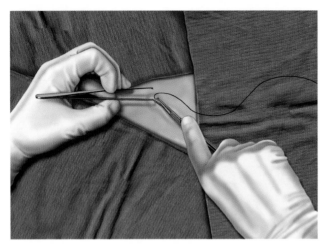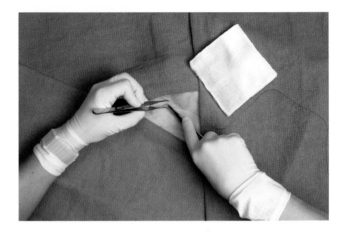

Step 1. Insert the needle close to the wound edge at a 90-degree angle to the skin surface.

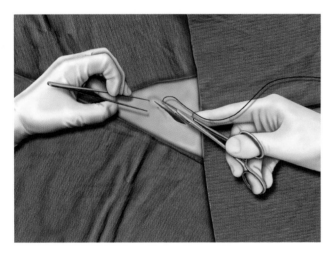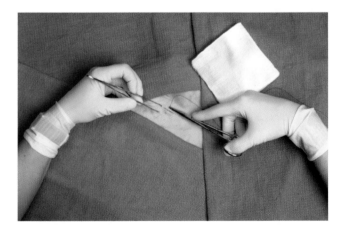

Step 2. Advance the needle in a circle approximating the shape of the needle toward the opposite side of the wound. Exit the wound on the opposite side close to the wound edge, at a 90-degree angle to the skin surface.

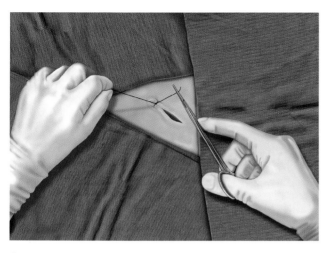 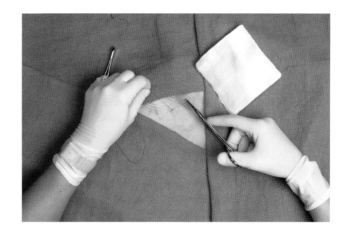

Step 3. Evert the edges of the wound and tie the suture with an instrument tie. Cut the ends of the suture.

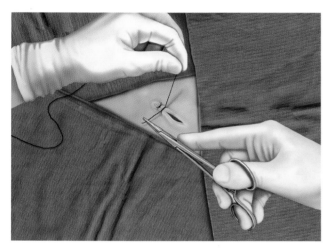 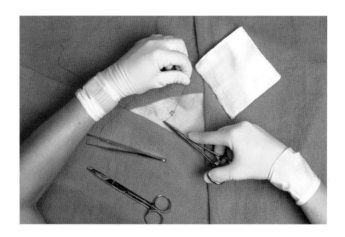

Step 4. Place subsequent sutures until the wound edges are apposed.

Continuous Suture

In the continuous suture technique, a continuous coil of sutures is placed through the skin with a knot at the two ends. Wound tension is more evenly distributed along the suture line because the suture is continuous rather than a series of separate sutures.

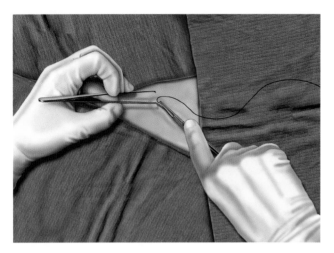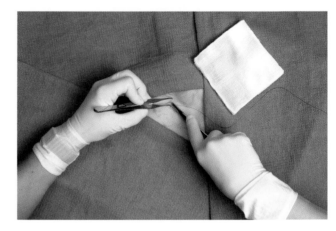

Step 1. Insert the needle close to the wound edge at a 90-degree angle to the skin surface.

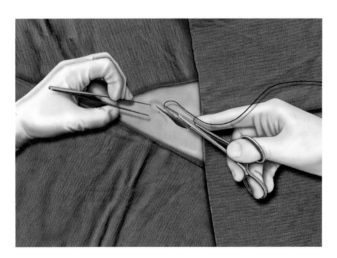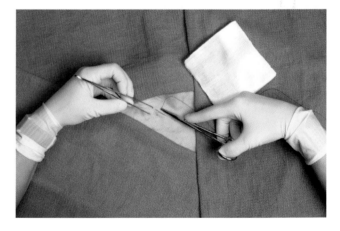

Step 2. Advance the needle in a circle approximating the shape of the needle toward the opposite side of the wound. Exit the wound on the opposite side close to the wound edge, at a 90-degree angle to the skin surface.

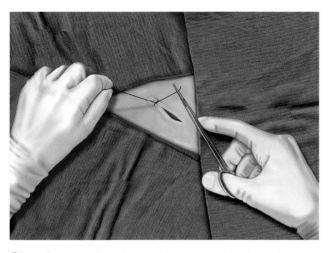 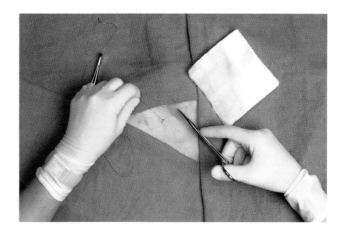

Step 3. Evert the edges of the wound and tie the suture with an instrument tie. Cut only the distal end of the suture, leaving the other end long and attached to the needle.

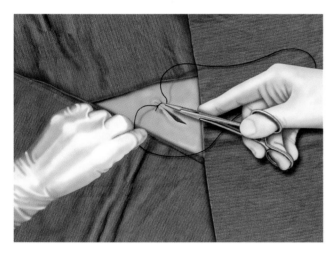 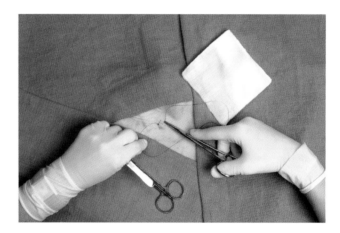

Step 4. Crossing over the wound to the opposite side at a 45-degree angle, re-enter the wound edge parallel to the original suture pass. Do not tie the suture or cut the ends.

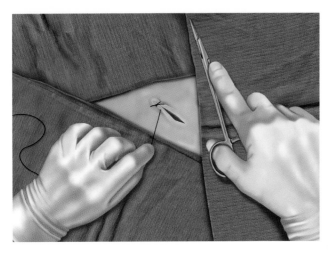 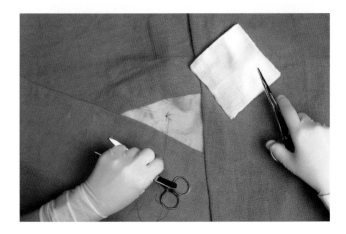

Step 5. Advance the needle back to the original side and exit the skin edge again at an equal distance from the previous suture pass.

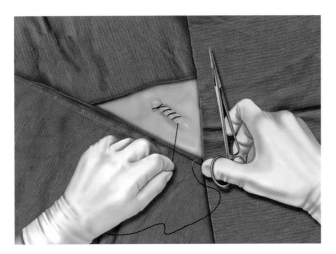 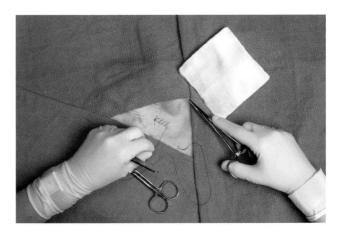

Step 6. In this fashion, continue to re-enter the skin until the wound edges are closed and the end of the wound is approached.

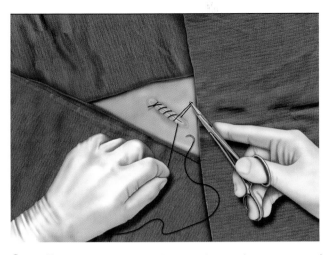 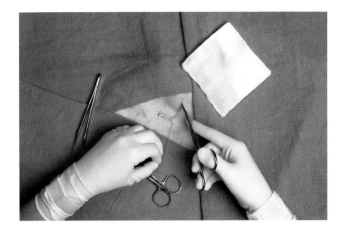

Step 7. On the last pass, leave a loop of suture. Use this loop as a free end to tie.

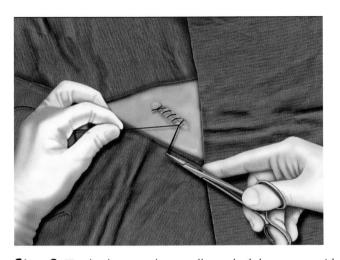 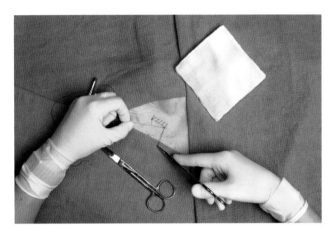

Step 8. Tie the loop to the needle end of the suture with an instrument tie.

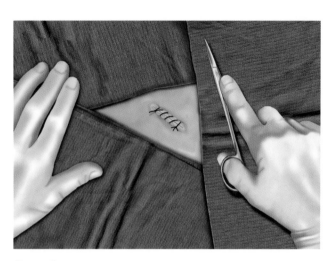 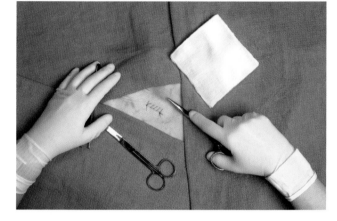

Step 9. Cut the loop and single ends of the suture.

Continuous Locked Suture

In the continuous suture technique, a continuous coil of sutures is placed in the skin with a knot at the two ends. Wound tension is evenly distributed along the suture line because the suture is continuous rather than a series of separate sutures. Locking the suture after each pass adds additional stability to the wound closure.

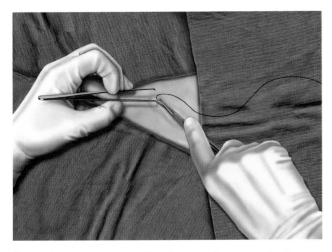

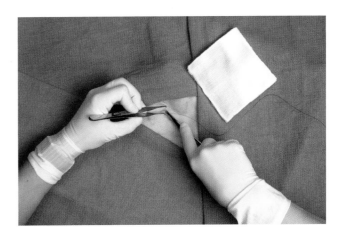

Step 1. Insert the needle close to the wound edge at a 90-degree angle to the skin surface.

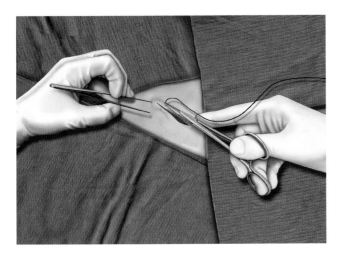

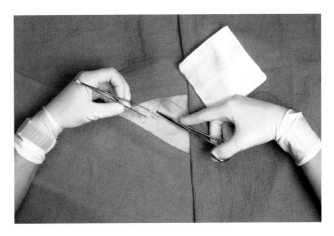

Step 2. Advance the needle in a circle approximating the shape of the needle toward the opposite side of the wound. Exit the wound on the opposite side, close to the wound edge, at a 90-degree angle to the skin surface.

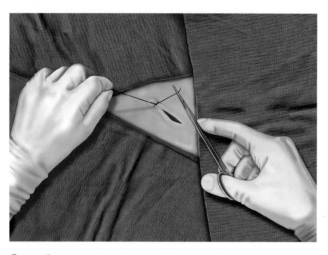
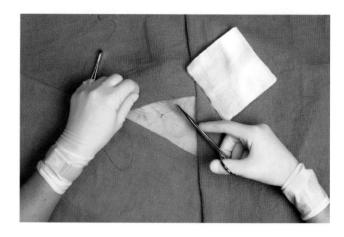

Step 3. Evert the edges of the wound and tie the suture with an instrument tie. Cut only the distal end of the suture, leaving the other end long and attached to the needle.

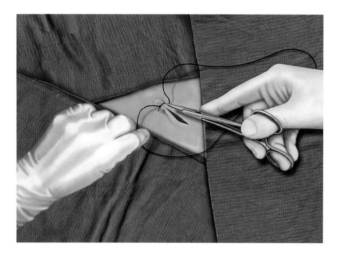
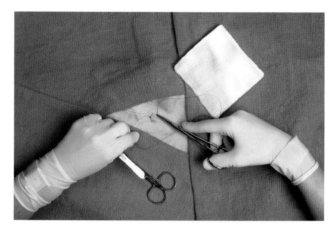

Step 4. Crossing over the wound to the opposite side at a 90-degree angle, re-enter the wound edge at a 90-degree angle and parallel to the original suture pass. Do not tie the suture or cut the ends.

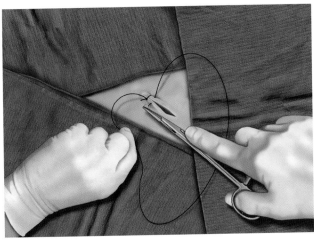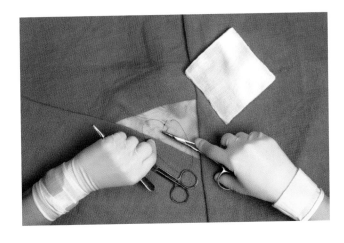

Step 5. Advance the needle back to the original side. Lock the suture by passing through the circle of the previous suture loop before exiting the skin edge at an equal distance from the previous suture pass.

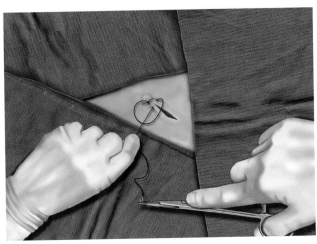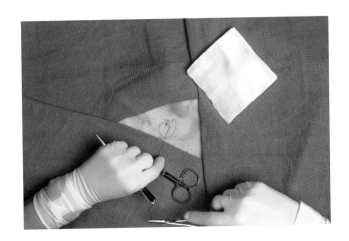

Step 6. As the suture is pulled through the circle, it will become locked.

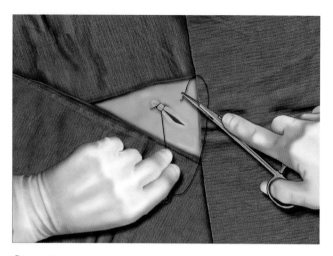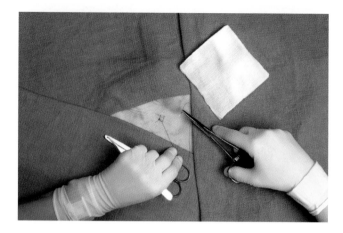

Step 7. Keep tension evenly distributed across the suture as it is pulled down to the skin.

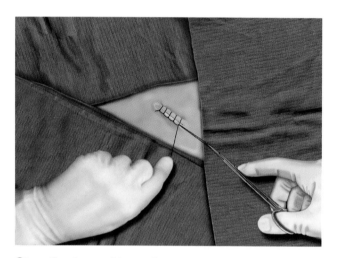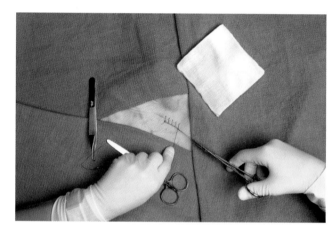

Step 8. Place additional sutures until the wound edges are closed. On the last pass, leave a loop of suture. Use this loop to function as a free end and tie it to the needle end of the suture with an instrument tie. Cut the ends of the suture.

Horizontal Mattress Suture

In the horizontal mattress suture technique, a second loop of suture is placed parallel and horizontal to the first in order to disperse the tension over the wound edges.

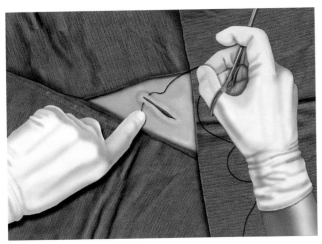
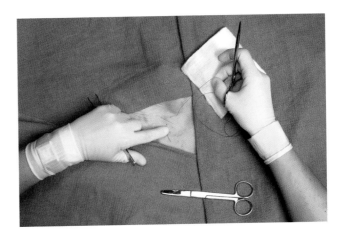

Step 1. Pass the needle through both sides of the wound in the same manner as the first pass in a simple interrupted suture.

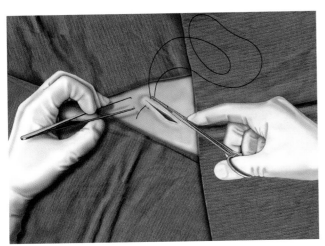
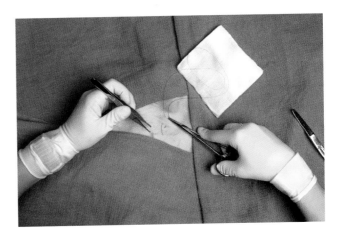

Step 2. Reinsert the needle approximately 0.5 cm from and horizontal to the previous exit site. Exit the wound on the opposite side parallel to the first pass and at the same distance from the wound edge.

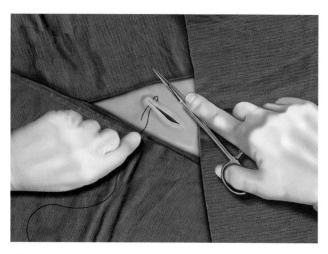
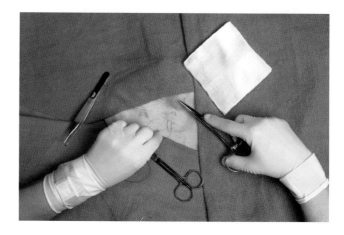

Step 3. Pull the suture through so that approximately 2 cm of the short end of the suture remains outside the skin.

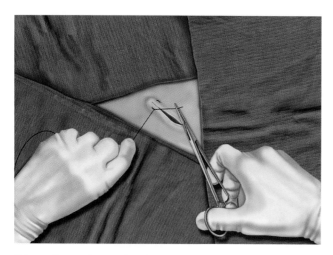
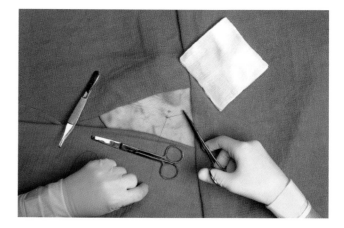

Step 4. Tie the ends of the suture with an instrument tie, while everting the edges of the wound. Cut the ends of the suture. Place subsequent sutures until the wound edges are apposed.

Vertical Mattress Suture

In the vertical mattress suture technique, a second loop of the suture is placed vertical to and deeper than the first in order to decrease tension on the wound edges.

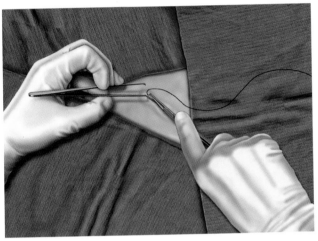 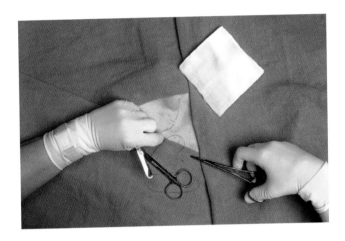

Step 1. Pass the needle through both sides of the wound in the same manner as the first pass in a simple interrupted suture.

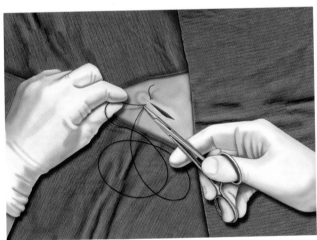 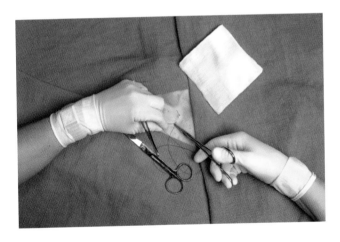

Step 2. Reinsert the needle vertical to the previous exit site at a greater distance from the wound edge.

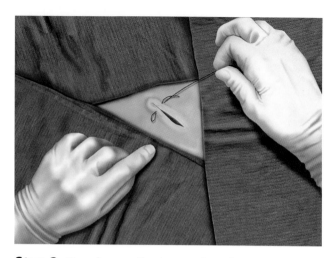 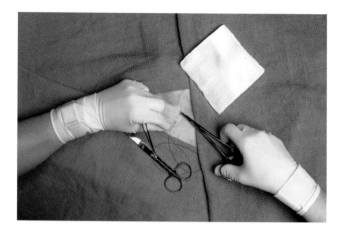

Step 3. Pass the needle deeper than the previous suture pass and exit the skin surface approximately 0.5 cm from and vertical to the previous entrance site. Pull the suture through so that approximately 2 cm of the short end of the suture remains outside the skin.

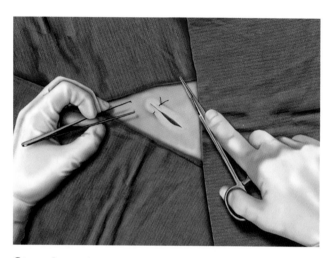 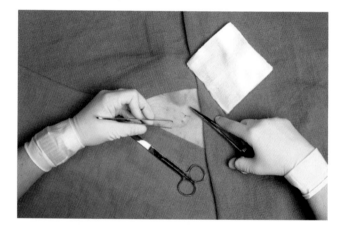

Step 4. Tie the ends of the suture with an instrument tie, while everting the edges of the wound. Cut the ends of the suture. Place subsequent sutures until the wound edges are apposed.

Deep Suture

In the deep suture technique, an absorbable intradermal suture is placed and the knot is buried deep to the dermis.

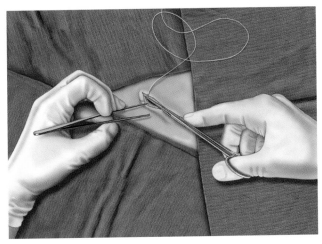

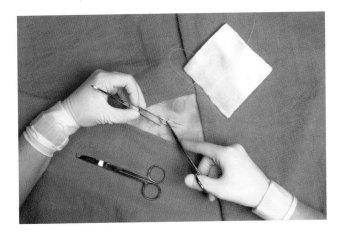

Step 1. Place the needle deep into the subcutaneous tissue at the wound edge. Advance the needle on the same side of the wound and exit at the level of the dermis with the needle parallel to the skin surface.

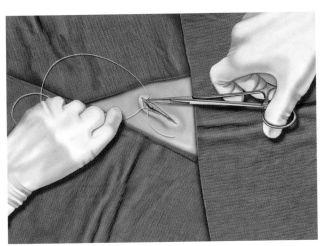

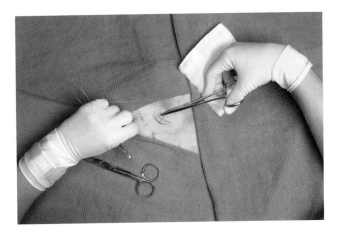

Step 2. On the opposite edge of the wound, place the needle into the dermis parallel to the skin surface and at the same distance as the suture on the opposite side. Advance the needle on the same side of the wound, exiting deep in the wound edge at the level of the subcutaneous tissue.

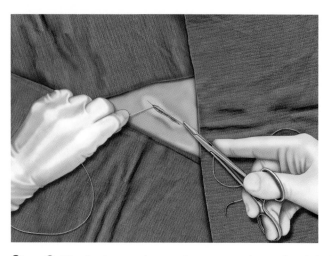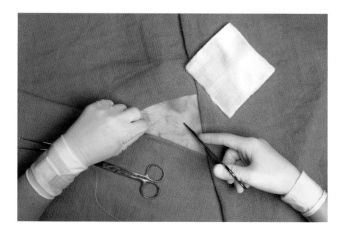

Step 3. Tie the knot using an instrument tie so that it is buried beneath the dermis.

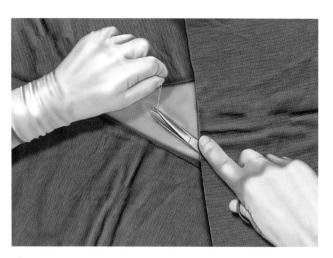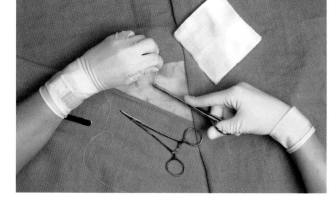

Step 4. Cut the suture ends close to the knot.

Staple Application

In the skin staple application technique, skin staples are applied across the edges of the wound to repair the laceration.

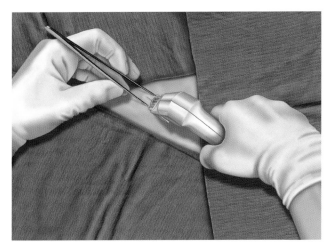

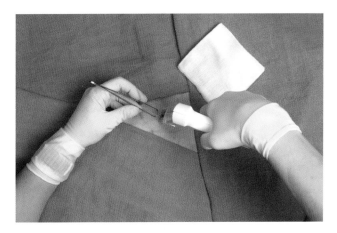

Step 1. Place the stapler perpendicular to the wound edge and at an equal distance from each side. Evert the edges of the wound. Squeeze and release the trigger of the stapler to bend the staple across the edges of the wound.

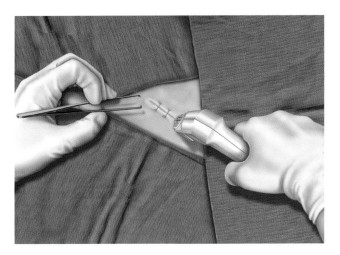

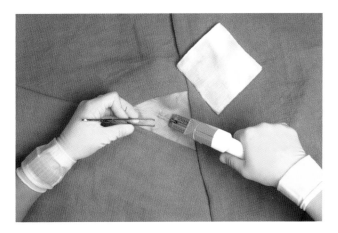

Step 2. Apply additional staples at equal distances until the wound edges are apposed.

Staple Removal

In the skin staple removal technique, skin staples are removed from the wound using a specialized device.

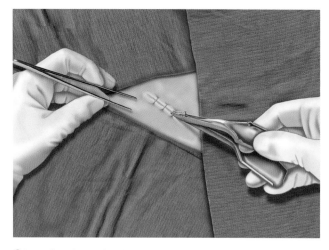

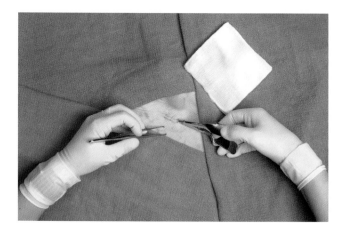

Step 1. Place the lower jaws (double parallel prongs) of the staple remover under the bottom of the staple and the upper jaw (single prong) over the top of the staple.

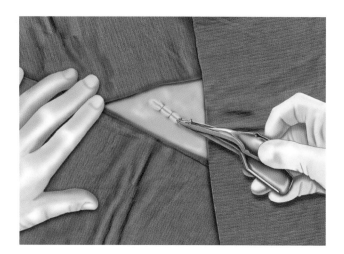

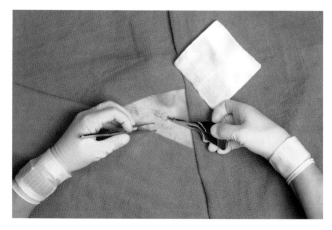

Step 2. Squeeze the handles of the staple remover to bend the staple open.

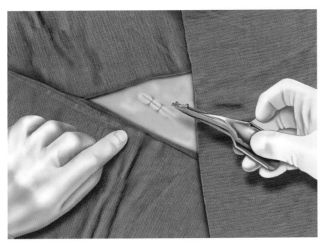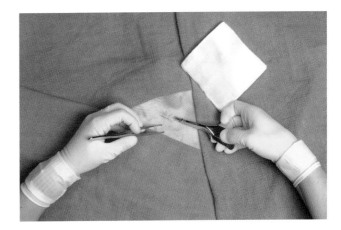

Step 3. Release the staple from the skin surface.

Wound Closure Tape Application

Wound closure tapes are adhesive strips applied across the edges of the wound to repair the laceration.

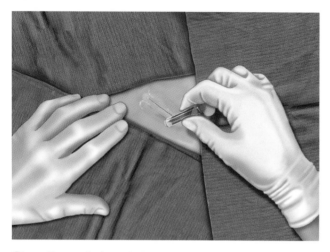 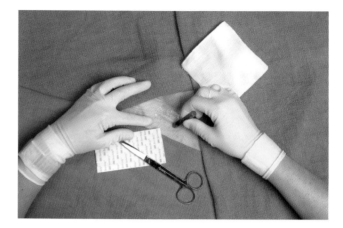

Step 1. Apply liquid skin adhesive, such as benzoin, parallel to the wound edges on both sides of the wound.

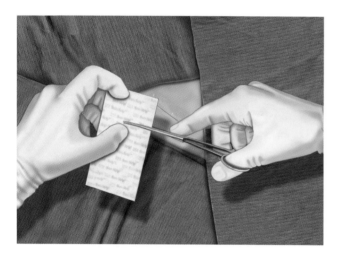 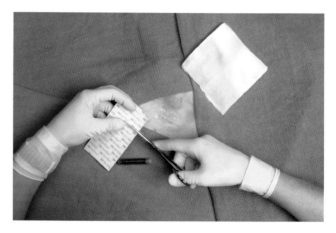

Step 2. Cut wound closure tape strips to a length sufficient to cover the wound edges on both sides.

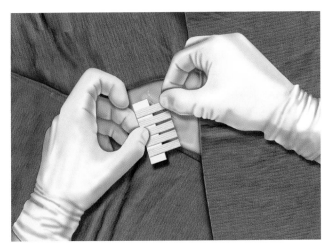
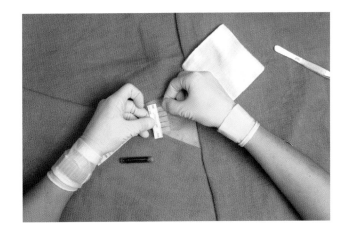

Step 3. Remove the wound closure tape strip from the paper backing.

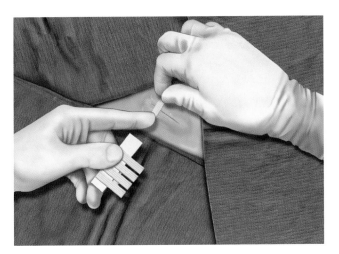
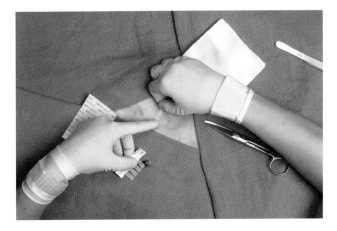

Step 4. Apply the wound closure tape strip to the skin perpendicular to the wound and covering an equal distance from each side of the wound.

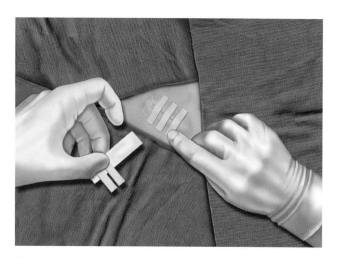 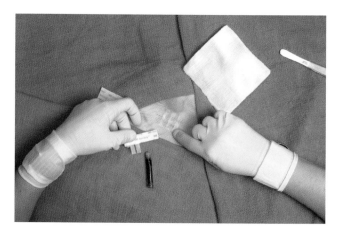

Step 5. Place additional wound closure tapes along the length of the wound until the wound edges are apposed.

Index